Administration for Exercise-Related Professions

Thomas D. Langley, EdD, JD

College of Charleston

Jerald D. Hawkins, EdD, ATC, FACSM

Lander University

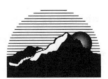

Morton Publishing Company
925 W. Kenyon Ave., Unit 12
Englewood, CO 80110
http://www.morton-pub.com

To our wives,

Janie and Sandra,

for their love, patience, encouragement, and support

TDL and JDH

The case scenarios presented in chapters 18-21 are based on actual events, but any resemblance to people and places is purely coincidental.

Printed in the United States of America
by Morton Publishing Company
925 W. Kenyon Ave., Unit 12, Englewood, CO 80110

10 9 8 7 6 5 4 3 2 1

ISBN: 0-89582-417-5

ABOUT THE AUTHORS

Thomas D. Langley, EdD, JD, is associate professor of Physical Education and Health at the College of Charleston, Charleston, South Carolina. He holds the Doctor of Education degree in Health Education Administration (1983) and the Juris Doctorate (1993), both from the University of South Carolina. Dr. Langley teaches courses in both physical education and health. His primary courses are History and Philosophy of Physical Education, Organization and Administration, and Legal Issues in Special Topics (including physical education and sport and health promotion).

In addition to his teaching, he has had experience in a wide variety of administrative positions, including serving as the first Executive Director of the South Carolina Governor's Physical Fitness Advisory Council, Director of Intramural Activities, Project Administrator for the Health Education Unit in a regional medical center, and Department Chair. He is a past president of the South Carolina Alliance for Health, Physical Education, Recreation and Dance and served for 13 years as department chair for physical education and health at both a private college and a public college.

In these positions, Dr. Langley's duties included program planning and administration, budget planning, program and personnel evaluation, facilities planning and management, equipment purchasing and management, teaching and advising, and maintenance and custodial work. He believes he learned the most about organization and administration as a maintenance man and custodian. After all, they hold the keys.

Jerald D. Hawkins, EdD, ATC, FACSM, is professor of Physical Education and Exercise Studies and Director of Sports Medicine Education at Lander University, Greenwood, South Carolina. A Fellow of the American College of Sports Medicine and National Athletic Trainers' Association certified athletic trainer, Dr. Hawkins holds the Doctor of Education Degree in Physical Education (Exercise Science) (1975) from the University of Georgia. In addition to his teaching and coaching experience in grades K–12, his college and university teaching has involved a wide variety of courses in physical education, health, sports medicine, exercise science, sport law, and administration.

Dr. Hawkins has served on the sports medicine staff at numerous national and international sports events including the 1990 Goodwill Games, World Junior Luge Championships, and U. S. Olympic Festivals, and was a college/university department chair for 13 years. He is the author of five books and many book chapters and articles, an active writer, speaker, and consultant in the areas of wellness, exercise science, legal issues in sport, and sports medicine. Dr. Hawkins was the recipient of the 1997–98 Lander University Distinguished Professor Award.

Acknowledgments

The authors express sincere appreciation to Doug Morton and the entire Morton Publishing family for their continued commitment to providing quality publications for the exercise-related professions, and to Joanne Saliger and Bob Schram for their wonderfully creative efforts in bringing this book to life.

The following people contributed case scenarios (Section V) which, we believe, have added a genuine touch of the real world to the book: Dr. Herb Appenzeller, Dr. Karen Austen, Dr. Lynne Gaskin, Mr. Charles Hershey, Mr. Bryan Madden, Dr. Susan Rozzi, Mr. Gene Sessoms, Mr. Van Taylor, and Dr. Kathy Tritschler. Thanks to each of you.

A special thank you to Karen Watson for her technical assistance in the preparation of the manuscript.

Finally, we are very grateful to our friends, colleagues, and students at the College of Charleston and Lander University, and to all the many others who contributed to the success of this project.

Contents

PART IV   LEGAL ISSUES IN EXERCISE-RELATED PROFESSIONS

PART V ADMINISTRATION IN SPECIFIC EXERCISE-RELATED PROFESSIONS: A CASE ANALYSIS APPROACH

Foreword

Sport administrators, professors of sport administration, and would-be administrators are searching for a text that will guide them to a successful career in one of the exercise-related professions. Many administration books emphasize theories, rules, formulas, and checklists, complete with statistical research. Because of the nature of human behavior, however, much of the material, though worthwhile, is quickly discarded by administrators when they are faced with real–life complex issues and problems. There has been a longstanding need for a hands–on text that offers a practical approach to administration, based on sound administrative and management theories, principles, and concepts. Tom Langley and Jerry Hawkins recognized this need. With their combined 62 years of experience in various aspects of education and sport, the authors have provided a text that skillfully integrates sound policies and procedures of administration with practical techniques for their successful utilization.

Administration For Exercise–Related Professions focuses on exercise–related professionals including physical educators, athletics directors, coaches, athletic trainers, fitness specialists, and intramural and recreational sport administrators. The text also provides a wealth of valuable information for *all administrators* who wish to develop the skills necessary for effective administration and leadership. This well-organized text is a virtual road map to successful administration, and a practical guidebook for any administrator. The mission of the text is clear — to combine theory and concepts with a strong concentration on practical strategies.

The chapters on the legal issues facing today's administrators in an ever-increasing litigious society (Section IV), reveal the authors' outstanding legal background. Langley, an attorney and able educator, and Hawkins, an experienced legal consultant and educator, use their experience to identify the legal issues of primary concern to administrators.

The five chapters in Section V, present open-ended scenarios submitted by administrators in physical education, athletics, sports medicine, adult fitness, and intramural and recreational sport. These case scenarios represent common, yet often complex, situations that actually occur daily and must be dealt with by administrators. They also provide the opportunity to think critically about strategies that may be employed to solve common administrative problems. They create excellent opportunities for group discussion and encourage the application of theories, concepts, and principles presented in the text. The issues found in these scenarios will be familiar to present administrators and will alert future administrators to similar situations they will confront in their professional roles.

The authors have written a text that fills a void in the fields of exercise-related administration and sport management. This outstanding resource sets a high standard for future books and is a perfect fit for professional preparation in the 21st century. I congratulate Tom Langley and Jerry Hawkins for recognizing the need for a comprehensive administration text and accepting the challenge of meeting that need by writing this book.

Herb Appenzeller, Ed.D.
Jefferson–Pilot Professor of
      Sport Management Emeritus
Guilford College

Historical Foundations

OBJECTIVES

After studying this chapter, you should be able to:

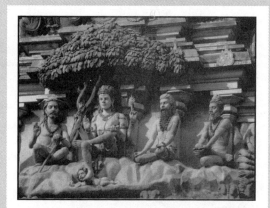

1. Identify the historical cultures that have influenced today's exercise-related professions and discuss the role of physical activity in each culture.

2. Identify the historical leaders who were instrumental in the development of sport and physical activity, and discuss the specific contributions of each.

3. Identify the historical events and leaders who have been instrumental in the development of the following exercise-related professions, and discuss the specific contributions of each:

   a. physical education
   b. athletics
   c. athletic training and sports medicine
   d. health promotion and adult fitness
   e. sport management
   f. recreation and intramural activities

From the dawn of civilization, physical activity has been an integral part of human daily activity. Ancient cave-wall etchings reveal that primitive people relied upon their physical skills to hunt and kill game and defend against predators, and running, jumping, and throwing were also an important part of social games play. As long as someone was known as a fast runner or a skilled jumper, someone has been willing to offer a challenge. In just such a setting the seeds of modern-day exercise and sport were planted.

CHINA (2700 BC)

Among the earliest known cultures to incorporate organized physical activity into the lifestyle were the ancient Chinese. Although ancient China was basically a isolationist nation, wrestling, soccer, polo, water games, and flying kites were popular activities. Based on their belief that physical inactivity can result in some types of disease, they used kneeling, bending, and stretching as forms of preventive and therapeutic exercise. Evidence indicates that Cong Fu (Chinese gymnastics) was practiced as early as 2700 B.C.

INDIA (2500 BC)

Similar to the Chinese, the ancient Indians were religious people whose Hindu beliefs led them to avoid glorification of the body and the accumulation of worldly goods. Despite these beliefs, however, the citizens of ancient India participated in activities such as tumbling, wrestling, running races, and dancing. Yoga — a formal program of postural and breathing exercises — was first practiced in ancient India.

NEAR EASTERN CULTURES (2000 BC)

Unlike their Chinese and Indian counterparts, the ancient Egyptians, Persians, and Syrians espoused a philosophy that life was to be enjoyed, including participation in a variety of physical activities. In addition to military training, which was known to be highly physical (wrestling, marching, archery, gymnastics, and the like), young Persians (boys age 6) were required to take part in horseback riding, hunting, javelin throwing, running, and similar activities deemed to be important for males.

ANCIENT GREECE (2500 BC – 400 AD)

Golden Age of Sport and Physical Education

Of all the ancient civilizations, none had a more dramatic influence on the historical development of exercise and sport than did ancient Greece. Because of this influence, the era has been called the Golden Age of Sport and Physical Education. The city-states of Athens and Sparta were the largest and most influential metropolitan centers of the ancient Greek world. Athens, with its philosophers, educators, and artists, was a cultural mecca, and Sparta was recognized as a powerful military training center.

Each, in its own unique way, played an important role in the historical development of exercise and sport.

Athens

The Athenian culture revolved around philosophical inquiry and artistic expression. The citizens of Athens also held a deep appreciation for the human body and often celebrated its beauty in drawings, sculptures, and writings (for example, Homer's *Iliad* and *Odyssey*) of the day. Philosophers and scientists such as Aristotle and Archimedes are recognized even today for their studies and subsequent writings concerning the mechanics of human movement.

Young Athenian males participated in "physical education" as a part of their daily education. In the *palaestra* (gymnasium-type buildings), young boys were instructed in methods of oiling and sanding the body by the *paidotribe* (physical education instructor), while older boys (14–16 years of age) were trained in the *gymnasia* (sport centers) by specialized coaches known as *gymnasts*. Contrary to today's common notion that intellectual prowess and athletic success are mutually exclusive concepts, the Athenians proclaimed that a complete person was one who possessed "a sound mind in a sound body."

Sparta

In direct contrast to Athens, Sparta's greatness was a result of its dedication to military excellence. Spartans were highly fit and militarily skilled. Consequently, the term *Spartan* has become synonymous with a lifestyle of rigorous physical and mental training. For this reason, many modern-day schools (including Michigan State University, University of Tampa, and San Jose State University) have chosen *Spartans* as the nickname for their athletic teams. In contrast, how many schools have adopted the nickname *Athenians* for their athletic teams?

Funeral Games

The ancient Greeks are well-known for their "funeral games" — sporting competitions organized and carried out in honor of the death of a revered Greek citizen. Funeral games often included contests of running, jumping, throwing, and weight lifting. These competitions provided an opportunity for towns, cities, and provinces to send their best athletes. The winners received the praise and adulation of their fellow citizens, in addition to the wreath of laurel or olive leaves that became symbolic of athletic excellence.

Funeral games

National Festivals

The widespread popularity of funeral games led to the organization of national sport festivals, which were early predecessors of the Olympic Games. These national festivals drew athletes from all parts of the known world. Although they were predominantly male-only events, occasional festivals were open to women and included musical activities. Winners at these festivals were often honored by their home cities with rather lavish gifts, prestigious jobs and housing, and celebrity status. Although the competitive philosophy of the ancient Greeks was rooted in the concept of amateurism (competition for the enjoyment of sport rather than for extrinsic rewards), athletes did move from city to city in response to more lucrative offers.

Birth of Olympic Games

Olympic Games An outgrowth of the national festivals, the first Olympic Games were held in 776 B.C. The original Olympic Games were held in tribute to the Greek god Zeus and featured competition in sports such as running, throwing, jumping, boxing, and wrestling. To compete, an athlete was required to meet several stringent requirements. The athlete had to

— be male

— train for a minimum of 10 months

— be a free man

— maintain a perfect physique and good moral character

— have no criminal record

— compete within the rules

— sign (along with his father, brothers, and trainer) the athletes' oath.

Once entered, the athlete was forced to compete, with no allowances for illness or injury.

The final requirement for Olympic Games was that all athletes, trainers, judges, and spectators had to take part in the nude. According to familiar legend, a young man was training under the direction of his father when, prior to the competition, his father died. With no other male trainers available, the athlete's mother assumed the role of trainer, and, to be able to accompany her son to the competition, disguised herself as a man. When she was discovered, officials decided to eliminate the possibility of future female intrusion into male-only games by requiring nude participation. The ancient Olympic Games were officially brought to an end by Roman law in 393 A.D., although the original ideals, values, and purposes of the Olympic Games had ceased to exist many years earlier.

Roman Empire (500 BC – 476 AD)

The rise to power of the Roman Empire was characterized by the world's first great military civilization. Every Roman citizen was expected to be prepared to go to battle if necessary. Thus the physical training of the "citizen-soldier" was an important aspect of Roman life. The early Roman philosophy was one of "all work and no play." As Rome's control of the known world grew, however, extravagant living, a love of luxury, and the pursuit of physical pleasure typified the Roman way of life.

In their unquenchable thirst for entertainment, Roman citizens turned away from participation in physical activity in favor of spectator sports. The carnal nature of the Roman Empire created a desire for sensational, often bloody, violent games. Fights between trained gladiator slaves became popular, with the winner often ordered to kill his opponent for the spectators' enjoyment.

In contrast to the "amateur" athletes of the early Roman Republic, athletes of the Roman Empire assumed the role of professionals. They were frequently bought and sold by cities in much the same way that professional athletes are traded today. Among the most famous athletes of the day was Diocles, a Spaniard who retired at age 42 having won more than 1,400 of the 4,200 races in which he competed. For his efforts, Diocles is believed to have won the equivalent of approximately $2 million during his career.

The Roman empire also gave birth to one of the world's first "sports medicine" specialists, a physician known as Galen. A Greek of Roman citizenship, Galen was one of the earliest known people to recognize and write about the health and therapeutic benefits of exercise and rest. It was under Roman rule that the Olympic Games were discontinued in 393 A.D.

Middle Ages (476 – 1600s AD)

Following the fall of the Roman Empire in 476, the world entered the turbulent period known as the Middle Ages. During this time Europe endured the Dark Ages, flourished in the Age of Feudalism, and celebrated cultural rebirth with the Age of Renaissance.

Dark Ages

In the years immediately following the Roman Empire's fall from power, Europe entered a period known as the Dark Ages. Little is known about

Christian asceticism

the specific details of life during this time. Except for the Teutonic armies' need for physical prowess so they could conquer their enemies, though, the Dark Ages represented a low point in sport and physical activity in Europe. One of the most influential forces in Europe during the Dark Ages was the Christian church, and its philosophy known as *Christian asceticism*. Simply stated, the prevailing belief was that the body and glorification of the body represented evil. Conversely, punishment of the body was considered an effective way to elevate the spirit and become more Godlike. As a result, clergy would seek ways to denigrate the body to gain spiritual favor. Church leaders commonly spent days and even weeks lying in caves while animals fed on their bodies, thereby allowing the spirit to be lifted closer to God, in their belief. Needless to say, exercise for the purpose of enjoyment or fitness was considered contrary to the will of God.

Scholasticism

The other major force in Europe at this time was *scholasticism*, the love of knowledge and intellectual development. Unlike the ancient Greeks, who espoused the philosophy that a sound mind and a sound body are inseparable, intellectuals of the Dark Ages sought to deemphasize physical development, believing that time spent in physical activity was time which could be better spent in intellectual pursuits.

Age of Feudalism

From the 9th to 14th centuries, Europe was governed largely by individual landowners who maintained military forces to defend the borders of their property. The king rewarded faithful noblemen by giving them large parcels of land to occupy and oversee in exchange for their protection from invading enemies. The landowners, in turn, awarded small tracts of the land to trusted allies in exchange for their military protection. Out of this system the often romanticized era of knights and ladies was born.

During the Age of Feudalism, physical training and formal education were available only to males. Consequently, most boys were either trained for work in the church or for knighthood. Knighthood training began at age 7 when a boy became a *page* serving as an errand boy and learning skills such as boxing, fencing, and swimming. At age 14 a page was elevated to *squire* status and was assigned to a specific knight for further training. A squire spent most his time perfecting the skills to be utilized in hunting, scaling walls, swordsmanship, and riding. Squires who proved themselves worthy were inducted into *knighthood* at age 21. The first responsibility of all knights was to provide protection against those who might invade and attempt to take over the land of their owners. Knights also participated in organized contests including jousting tournaments, in which losers frequently died as a result of the wounds they incurred in the competition.

Renaissance

As the name implies, the Renaissance period was a time of unparalleled cultural rebirth. Although this period is most often associated with art and music, the Renaissance was also a time of rebirth of appreciation of the many values of physical activity. Among the ideas that characterized this period were the unity of the body, mind, and spirit, the relationship of physical health and learning, and the benefits of rest and recreational activities to relieve the stress of studies and work.

Many noted church leaders, writers, philosophers, and educators of the Renaissance period spoke and wrote openly of the need for physical education (they, of course, did not use that term).

- In Italy, educator Vittorino da Feltra was among the first to combine physical and mental training by including daily physical activity in the school curriculum.

- Pope Pius II stated that physical activity contributes to good posture, total body health, and learning.

- German church leader Martin Luther saw physical activity as a desirable substitute for "leisure vices" as well as a way of maintaining health.

- French theorist Francois Rabelais wrote that regular physical activity was an important part of education because of its ability to facilitate mental development.

- English poet John Milton wrote that exercise was valuable for both bodily development and preparation for war.

This newfound enthusiasm for physical activity demonstrated that the Renaissance was not only cultural but physical as well.

EUROPE (MID 1700s – LATE 1800s)

By the mid 1700s, physical activity and sport had attained more respect throughout Europe. Throughout the following century (a period often referred to as the Age of Nationalism), several European nations (primarily Germany, Sweden, England, and France) undertook the development of formal physical education and sports programs, which have had a direct influence on contemporary physical education, sport, and other exercise-related professions.

Germany

The modern world's first nationalistic power was Germany. The German people adopted a national commitment to a lifestyle of rigid discipline in the belief that a nation is no stronger than its citizens and, through this strength, a nation could best protect its independence. Out of this philosophy grew the formal system of rigorous, regimented exercise that would come to be known as *German Gymnastics*. Unlike modern-day gymnastics, the German system included activities such as synchronized marching and rigid adherence to postural alignment. Some names of note are the following.

- Johann Basedow, a German education reformer, founded the first school in modern Europe to include physical education in the school curriculum.

- Johann Cristoph Guts Muths, a physical educator, wrote the first book on German gymnastics, *Gymnastics for the Young*, in 1793.

- Friedrich Ludwig Jahn, a contemporary of Guts Muths, believed that physical training through gymnastics was the best way for Germany to remain a strong, independent nation and founded a society of gymnasts known as the *Turnverein*. The proliferation of Turnverein Societies throughout Germany became know as the *Turnverein Movement*. At the peak of the *Turnverein Movement*, several years after Jahn's death, there were more than 10,000 Turnverein Societies, some of which are still in place today.

- Adolph Spiess, a student of Turnverein gymnastics, espoused a *total person* educational philosophy and recommended that every young person, boys and girls alike, should have 1 hour of physical education instruction every day with grades awarded according to achievement. His 1828 book, *Manual of Gymnastics* was adopted as the curriculum guide for German schools. He was possibly the most important figure in the development of school gymnastics.

Turnverein

Sweden

Germany was not the only nation experiencing patriotic fervor during this time. Having lost territorial disputes with Russia, Sweden called upon its citizens to be prepared to protect and preserve Sweden's heritage. The following were instrumental in the development of physical education.

- Per Henrik Ling, a student of Scandinavian culture, founded the Royal Central Institute of Gymnastics in Stockholm, where instructors were required to have an understanding of human anatomy and physiology and exercise physiology, primitive though it was. Prior to Ling's work, the value of physical activity had been based largely on the apparent benefits to the body, although the benefits were not supported by good scientific research. Ling believed that the study of physical education should be rooted in sound, scientific reasoning.

- Lars Gabriel Branting, a protege of Ling, expanded the study of exercise anatomy and physiology to include the cardiovascular, respiratory, and nervous systems. His main interest was in what was known as *medical gymnastics*, the therapeutic aspects of exercise.

- Gustaf Nyblaes, a military gymnastics enthusiast, was Branting's successor as director of the Royal Central Institute of Gymnastics. Under his leadership of Nyblaes women were first admitted for study at the Royal Institute.

Britain

Britain may be called the birthplace of outdoor sports. As early as the 14th century, there is evidence of a game similar to tennis being played in England. Other outdoor games that are rooted in Britain include golf (as early as 1600 in Scotland) and cricket (as early as 1700 in England). One of the most notable names in the history of British sport and physical education was Archibald McLaren, who applied medical concepts to the teaching of physical education and sport. He believed, as did the ancient Greeks, that the mind and body are inseparable. His work included designing a system of physical training for the British military.

France

Although not a world leader in the same manner as Germany, Sweden, and England, France played a significant role in the development of physical education and sport. Three names are of special note.

- Jean-Jacques Rousseau, a proponent of education reform in Europe, was one of the first people to challenge the church's position of avoiding play, or leisure activity. His unpopular position resulted in his imprisonment.

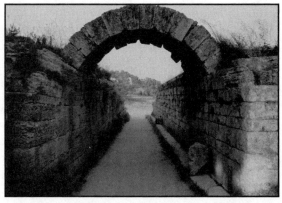

Entrance to the Original Olympic Stadium, Olympia, Greece.

- Johann Basedow's interest in the value of physical activity in the schools was stimulated by Rousseau's book *Emile*.

- Baron Pierre de Coubertin led the effort to revive the Olympic Games, which had been abolished by Roman decree in the year 393 A.D. As a direct result of his efforts, the first games of the Modern Olympiad were held in Athens, Greece, in 1893.

UNITED STATES

The history of American sport and physical education goes back to the arrival of the first settlers in the new world in the early 1600s.

Colonial America (early 1600s–late 1700s)

Colonial America was divided into three distinct segments, each with its own influence on the physical activity practices in the new land.

1. The *New England colonies* were established primarily by English dissidents who left their homeland in search of religious freedom. Most of the original colonists held strict, puritanical religious beliefs — thus the name by which they were known, Puritans. One of the tenets the colonists shared was that pleasure was surely a device of the devil and to be avoided at all costs. Therefore, physical activity that brought enjoyment or benefited the body was looked down upon, and those who engaged in physical activity other than work were often severely punished for their transgressions.

2. Just below the original colonies was *an area bordering the Hudson River*, today known as New York. The early settlers of this land were primarily of Dutch descent. Unlike their neighbors to the north, the Dutch settlers enjoyed physical activity and made ice skating, coasting (sledding), and hunting a regular part of their lifestyle.

3. The third segment of colonial America lay *south of the Dutch settlements*, now known as the Carolinas, Georgia, Tennessee, Alabama, and Kentucky. It was populated largely by English prisoners and malcontents. During the settlement of the New England colonies, Spaniards and others who were entering the new world from the south in their quest for gold frequently attacked the settlements. When England received word of this newfound threat to the colonies, it rejected the request for military intervention and instead offered to release inmates from debtors' prisons along with other minor criminals in exchange for their agreement to be

shipped to the new world to protect the colonies from the southern invasions. With little to lose, many English citizens agreed to a new life in the southern part of the new world. It is from these early settlers physical activities such as dancing, boxing, horse racing, cock fights, and cricket found their way into colonial America.

Nationalist America (late 1700s–Civil War)

Following the American Revolution of the late 1700s, the colonists' attention turned to the business of constructing the world's newest nation. One of the major concerns was that of establishing an effective system of education for America's youth. Early academies, the equivalent of secondary schools, emphasized instruction in the traditional *3Rs* — reading, writing, and math. Little opportunity was available for physical activity, although after-school games and sports were popular with many students. In 1802 the U.S. government established the United States Military Academy at West Point, which included a strong emphasis on physical training.

During the next decade Europeans immigrating to America brought with them the influence of Jahn's German Gymnastics. The first American school to include instruction in formal gymnastics was the Round Hill School in Northampton, Massachusetts, founded by Charles Beck in 1823. In nearby Boston, Charles Follen became the first university instructor of gymnastics in the United States. Despite the efforts of Beck and Follen, early attempts to incorporate gymnastics into America's schools were generally unsuccessful.

By the mid-1800s, the Turnverein influence was taking hold in the northeastern part of America. By the 1850s there were nearly two dozen active Turnverein Societies, the oldest of which was established in Cincinnati in 1848 and remains to this day. During this period Catherine Beecher established the first formal exercise program for women at the Hartford Female Seminary. In addition to these specific events of the pre-Civil War era, gymnasium buildings began to spring up as Swedish gymnastics achieved popularity and colleges and universities formed gymnastics clubs.

Post-Civil War America (Civil War–1900)

With the end of the Civil War came a period of social reconstruction, including increased interest in making physical activity an integral part of education. Turnverein groups for boys and girls alike became popular, and exercise programs focused on the health benefits of regular physical

Normal school

activity. One of the leading figures in the movement toward school-based physical education was Dr. Dio Lewis, who, in 1861 established the nation's first *normal school* (teacher preparation school) in Boston for the training of physical education teachers. Ling-style gymnastics grew in popularity, resulting in the founding of the Swedish Health Institute in Washington, DC by Hartvig Nissen.

HISTORY OF EXERCISE-RELATED PROFESSIONS IN THE UNITED STATES

Most, if not all, of the exercise-related professions share a common history prior to the 20th century. In recent years, however, the desire for specialization in all fields of endeavor has led to the development of a myriad of specific exercise-related professions, each with its own, albeit it young, history.

Physical Education and Athletics

In the late 1800s, two major characteristics typified physical education and athletics in the United States: tremendous growth in popularity and little distinction between the two in the public view — a concern that exists even today. As early as 1866, an attempt was made to require physical education as a part of the school curriculum when California mandated 5 minutes of exercise daily as a part of the prescribed school day. This mandate was short-lived, however, and required physical education did not become a permanent fixture in the school curriculum until such a law was passed in Ohio in 1892. One year later, in 1893, Harvard College, now Harvard University — a contemporary bastion of intellectual inquiry — granted the nation's first college degree in physical education.

Although physical education approached the turn of the 20th century with increased interest and popularity, its growth was threatened by what has been aptly called the "battle of the systems." As discussed earlier, both the German and Swedish systems of exercise had large followings, so the issue of which system would ultimately serve as foundation for the development of a nationwide physical education philosophy was a topic of heated debate.

In response to the debate over a national system of physical education, Dudley Sargent, professor of physical education at Harvard, introduced his system of exercise and established the Sargent Normal School in 1881. The current Sargent School of Allied Health Sciences at Boston University is the product of Sargent's original efforts to create a system characterized by a blending of both the theoretical and the practical study of exercise. In 1885, American physical educators united to form the Association for the Advancement of Physical Education. The first professional organization for physical educators in the United States, the AAPE elected Edward Hitchcock of Amherst College its first president. After numerous name changes and tremendous expansion in the types of professions represented in its membership, this organization is known today as the American Alliance for Health, Physical Education, Recreation and Dance. AAHPERD is America's largest physical education-related organization.

The evolution of physical education in the 20th century was influenced by leaders such as Sargent, Hitchcock, Jessie Bancroft, Thomas Wood, Clark Hetherington, R. Tait McKenzie, Delphine Hanna, Jay B. Nash, Jesse Feiring Williams, Charles McCloy, Rosalind Cassidy, Eleanor Metheny, and Luther Gulick. For a detailed discussion of the roles of these and other prominent figures, the reader is encouraged to consult *Physical Education and Sport: A Contemporary Introduction* (1994), by Angela Lumpkin.

Contemporary physical education in America bears only a slight resemblance to the German and Swedish systems from which it emanated. A nationwide concern over the apparent apathy of American citizens toward the physical well-being of our children, as well as adults, is clearly shown in *America 2000: An Education Strategy*. Released in 1991, this document provides a comprehensive look at the present status and future of education in the United States. Although a wide range of philosophies still guide the development of American physical education, many contemporary physical educators agree that the aim of physical education should be to create efficient and effective movers who will choose to be physically active for a lifetime.

The mid-19th century to the present has also seen a dramatic growth in the area of competitive sports or athletics. Some of the more notable events in athletics prior to the turn of the 20th century are presented in Table 1.1.

There has been an unparalleled explosion of popularity of competitive sports in the United States in the 20th century. From youth sports for children as young as 4 years of age to professional sports, athletics has become a major social and economic force in contemporary society. Today, collegiate and professional athletes and coaches routinely perform before thousands of spectators, generating billions of dollars for the support of a variety of collegiate programs, salaries for college and professional coaches, and salaries for professional athletes — salaries that often surpass those of the CEOs of our nation's leading companies. The public influence of professional athletes rivals that of the most famous and highest paid entertainers and is often greater than that of elected officials.

TABLE 1.1   *Pre-20th Century Events in Athletics*

Date	Event	Sponsor/Initiator
1852	First collegiate sports contest	Crew race, Harvard d. Yale
1859	First baseball game	Amherst d. Williams, 73–32
1869	First football game	Rutgers d. Princeton, 6–4
1874	Tennis brought to America from Bermuda	Mary Outerbridge
1877	First lacrosse game	New York University d. Manhattan, 2–0
1891	Invention of basketball	Dr. James Naismith, Springfield, MA YMCA
1895	Invention of volleyball	William Morgan, Holyoke, MA YMCA
1896	First collegiate sports contest for women (basketball)	Stanford d. California, 2–1

Athletic Training and Sports Medicine

As with physical education and sport, the professions of athletic training and sports medicine can be traced back to the beginning of recorded history. As long as athletes have engaged in competition, they have suffered injuries for which they needed care and have looked for ways to improve performance beyond simply engaging in physical training. Thus, the need for athletic trainers and sports medicine specialists has always existed. As far back as the Golden Age of Greece, records show people serving as sports medicine assistants to athletes. For injury prevention and care, the standard approach was usually a combination of massage and herbal remedies. Primitive attempts at improving performance involved practices such as drinking deer blood to improve running speed and drinking beverages to which powdered lions' teeth had been added to enhance strength and courage, since deer were fast animals, and lions were the epitome of courage). These are but two examples of the common (though erroneous) conclusions to which primitive athletes often jumped.

Although physicians often volunteered their expertise to assist athletes and athletic teams, U. S. athletic training and sports medicine can be most directly traced to the late 19th century. The development and proliferation of collegiate and professional sports in the United States spawned a new classification of sports enthusiast. These people loved sports and yet were unable to participate, so they assumed the role of athletic trainer, thereby allowing them to be a part of a sports team, albeit an unofficial part. These individuals were basically hangers-on with little or no qualifications and often questionable backgrounds. Their services consisted mainly of providing rub-downs for players.

Because of their lack of knowledge and skill, athletic training and sports medicine were accepted slowly. The 1950s ushered in the modern age of athletic training and sports medicine, with the founding of the two largest professional organizations for athletic trainers and sports medicine professionals. In 1950, the National Athletic Trainers' Association (NATA) was established and today is the driving force behind athletic training in the United States. The standard of professional recognition for an athletic trainer is certification by the NATA. In 1954, the American College of Sports Medicine (ACSM) was founded and continues to be the largest professional organization for sports medicine professionals in the world. ACSM also offers certification programs at various levels of preventive and rehabilitative exercise programming.

Health Promotion and Adult Fitness

Health promotion — often called *wellness* — and adult fitness are relatively young professions that represent a merging of the concerns and utilization of knowledge from the fields of health, physical fitness, and exercise science. Dr. Dudley Sargent began his quest for optimal fitness for all Americans at Harvard in 1879. His program of individualized exercise prescriptions and physical training was designed to improve the structural and functional quality of life. Subsequently, the most obvious driving force behind America's "on again/off again" interest in physical fitness has been U. S. involvement in war. With each military encounter, concern for the health and fitness of U.S. youth grew, and with each successive time of peace and prosperity, the concern waned.

Two major events of the 1950s, however, stimulated the interest in physical fitness that exists today.

1. Autopsy studies of young men and women killed in the Korean war revealed that, despite their youth, at least 70% of them had signs of significant coronary artery disease.

2. Research conducted by Dr. Hans Kraus indicated that U.S. youth performed poorly on tests of muscular function when compared to European youth.

Concern over these findings led President Dwight D. Eisenhower to establish the President's Council on Youth Fitness in 1955. During the presidency of John F. Kennedy, the name of this council was changed to the President's Council on Physical Fitness, and again to the President's Council on Physical Fitness and Sports by President Richard M. Nixon. Under the direction of this council, the *Youth Fitness Test* was developed, the predecessor to subsequent health-related fitness tests such as AAHPERD's *Physical Best* and the current *FitnessGram*, developed by the Cooper Institute for Aerobics Research.

No single person has had a more profound impact on health promotion and fitness in the United States than Dr. Kenneth Cooper, a former Air Force physician who could rightly be called the "father of aerobics." Research on thousands of subjects convinced Cooper that our greatest fitness need was regular participation in aerobic activity. Cooper's first book, *Aerobics*, published in 1967, introduced the concept of aerobic exercise and its benefits in a practical, yet scientifically sound manner. Under his leadership, the Cooper Institute for Aerobic Research in Dallas, Texas, has become one of the largest and most prestigious research and adult fitness centers in the world.

No field of exercise science has had a more direct and significant influence on modern U.S. health promotion and adult fitness than that of exercise physiology. Research on the specific ways in which the human body adapts to physical activity has been the very foundation for development of sound health promotion and adult fitness programs. The roots of modern exercise physiology can be traced to the contributions of three European scientists.

- A. V. Hill, a pioneer in the study of aerobic performance, coined the term "maximal oxygen intake" in 1924.
- August Krogh's early work paved the way for today's sophisticated knowledge of capillary circulation.
- Otto Meyerhof was one of the first to study the relationship of glucose metabolism, lactic acid formation, and fatigue.

In recognition of their contributions to the advancement of scientific knowledge, each of these three exercise physiologists received the prestigious Nobel Prize.

Most authorities agree that the single most important influence on the evolution of exercise physiology in the United States was the Harvard Fatigue Laboratory (1927–1947) under the direction of Dr. David Bruce Dill. The first comprehensive exercise physiology research center in the United States, it drew doctoral students and research scientists from around the world and became the model for exercise and environmental research. Much of the research conducted at the Harvard Fatigue Lab is recognized even today for its excellence, precision, and influence on contemporary exercise physiology.

Sport Management

Although sport management did not come into its own as a profession until the latter part of the 20th century, it is believed that even among the ancient Greeks were individuals who took responsibility for the management of sporting events. Therefore, it can be argued that sport management has a long history. The birthplace of modern sport management, however, is considered to be Ohio University in Athens, Ohio, where Dr. James Mason designed the first sport management academic curriculum in 1967. Even though contemporary sport management professionals are typically graduates of formal undergraduate or graduate sport management programs, the public has been slow to accept the management of sport in the same way as it does management in industry. The major reason for this may be the prevailing attitude that sport is generally associated with play, whereas management is associated with work. In addition to Mason, others who were instrumental in the development and emergence of sport management in America are Dr. Guy Lewis (University of Massachusetts), Dr. Herb Appenzeller (Guilford College), Dr. Joy Sidwell (Bowling Green State University), Dr. Michael Ritchey (Warsaw Professional Sport Marketing program, University of Oregon), Dr. Wayne Blann (Ithaca College) and Dr. Stan Brassie (University of Georgia).

Recreation and Intramural Activities

Recreational and leisure activities certainly are among the oldest forms of human physical activity. Virtually all of the activities that have become part of the competitive world of athletics originated for pure enjoyment. Therefore, the early history of recreational and leisure activity is inseparably interwoven with that of sport.

By the mid-19th century Americans were seeking opportunities for physical activity outside the rigid environment of gymnastics and the competitive venues of sports. The founding of the Young Men's Christian Association (YMCA) in 1851 and the Young Women's Christian Association (YWCA) in 1866 offered physical activity (educational, competitive, and recreational) for many people. In 1906, the Playground Association of America was founded, and later changed its name to the National Recreation and Parks Association (NRPA), the nation's largest professional organization for recreation professionals. Today, recreation, or leisure activity is recognized as the nation's largest industry as measured by consumer spending.

Prior to the 1950s, professional preparation programs in recreation focused on training students how to manage recreational programs in non-school settings. In 1950, the National Intramural Association was founded by Dr. William Wasson for professionals working in college and university intramural sports programs. In 1975, in recognition of the organization's expanded and diversified role, the membership voted to change its name to the National Intramural-Recreational Sport Association (NIRSA). Currently several schools offer professional preparation degree programs in intramural and recreational sport administration.

RESOURCES

Arnheim, D.D. & Prentice W.E. (1997). *Principles of Athletic Training*, 9th ed. Dubuque, IA: Brown & Benchmark Publishers.

Hawkins, J. D. (1993). *The Practical Delivery of Sports Medicine Services: A Conceptual Approach*. Canton, OH: PRC Publishing.

Lewis, G. & Appenzeller, H. (1985). *Successful Sport Management*. Charlottesville, VA: Michie Co.

Lumpkin, A. (1994). *Physical Education and Sport: A Contemporary Introduction*, 3d ed. St. Louis: Mosby-Year Book.

Mull, R. F., Bayless, K. G. & Craig, M. R. (1987). *Recreational Sports Programming: Sports for All*, 2d ed. North Palm Beach, FL: Athletic Institute.

Powers, S.K. & Howley, E.T. (1997). *Exercise Physiology: Theory and Application to Fitness and Performance*, 3d ed. Dubuque, IA: Brown & Benchmark Publishers.

Siedentop, D. (1998). *Introduction to Physical Education, Fitness, and Sport*, 3d ed. Mountain View, CA: Mayfield Publishing.

Wuest, D. A. & Bucher, C. A. (1995). *Foundations of Physical Education and Sport*, 12th ed. St. Louis: Mosby-Year Book.

Contemporary Trends and Issues

After studying this chapter, you should be able to:

1. Identify and discuss at least five current trends in the exercise-related professions.

2. Discuss an issue associated with any of the trends listed in #1 above.

3. Identify a trend that could serve as a "common goal" for all exercise-related professions.

4. Identify two trends associated with professional development, and discuss the potential impact of each on program planning in the profession.

5. Discuss the relationship between the trends of privatization of leisure and those of lack of availability of activity opportunities based on socioeconomic status and age.

6. Discuss the effect the trend of "pay for play" in public recreation might have on the availability of activity opportunities.

7. Discuss the potential impact the quality of physical education programs and the exclusionary practices of varsity athletics might have on attitudes toward lifelong physical activity.

8. Identify the concerns related to equity in sport in relation to participation and employment.

9. Given any trend, discuss a potential impact on programming or personnel.

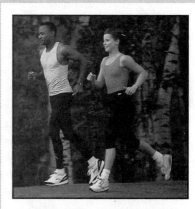

rends and issues cannot be neatly separated into a list of trends and a list of issues. This is primarily the case because one person's trend is another person's issue. Also, some trends are controversial and, as a result, become issues. Even those that are not controversial might raise issues for some people while others see no issues involved. With that said, below is a discussion of trends *and* issues gleaned from recent literature, including the effect these trends and issues might have on management in the exercise-related professions.

COMMON GOALS
FOR EXERCISE-RELATED PROFESSIONALS

People outside the profession are becoming increasingly aware of the positive health benefits to be gained from life-long physical activity, and those inside the profession are coming to realize that the various exercise-related professions must work together if the profession is to help everyone realize these benefits. Even though this common goal for the exercise-related professions seems laudable, it raises issues of loss of autonomy for individual segments of the profession and of developing links among the various segments that everyone can support.

*Hypokinetic
diseases*

With the publication of the Surgeon General's Report on Physical Activity and Health in 1996, what has been common knowledge to people in the exercise-related professions for some time was presented to the American public. This common knowledge is that participation in moderate physical activity in general and in fitness-enhancing activity in particular results in multiple health benefits. This is particularly true in relation to the chronic, or *hypokinetic*, diseases that plague society today — diseases such as coronary heart disease, hypertension, osteoporosis, noninsulin-dependent diabetes, chronic back pain, and obesity.

Steve Blair of the Cooper Aerobic Institute in Dallas, Texas, a major author of the Surgeon General's report, likened the 1996 report to the 1964 Surgeon General's report on *Smoking and Health*. Blair observed that when the 1964 report was first published, people took note of it, but a concentrated effort over 30 years has been necessary to reap the benefits of that report. The 1996 report is the first step in a journey that will require another concentrated effort from people in the exercise-related professions to reach its destination. Those of us in the exercise-related professions, particularly those in administrative positions, have to provide programs and personnel that will make the trip a successful one.

*Lifespan physical
activity*

Persons can become involved in purposeful physical activity very early in life and can continue to pursue these interests throughout their lives (lifespan physical activity). Unfortunately, that possibility has not yet been realized for many people. . . .

Someday, historians will describe the current era as a watershed period characterized by the emergence of the possibility for lifespan physical activity — in sport, fitness, and physical education. We have not yet achieved lifespan physical activity, but we now know that it is both possible and desirable. What we have to do now is to create the opportunity to achieve it.

Daryl Siedentop, 1998

Most authors writing on trends and issues in physical education acknowledge the need for all exercise-related professionals to recognize the role they play, or can play, in encouraging U. S. citizens to be active throughout life. The quote by Siedentop above is representative of this awareness and calls all exercise-related professionals to take part in creating an environment that will encourage, and allow, all citizens to be active.

This issue is highly relevant to the topic of management. It points to the development of common goals for all exercise-related professions. At a minimum, this would involve setting a goal of creating an opportunity for individuals of all ages to be involved in physical activity and a goal of ensuring that individuals can and will take advantage of this opportunity to move toward a state of wellness.

Setting and meeting these goals is a major management consideration. Administrators would have to consider new programs. They would have to determine whether these changes would require a major change in current programming or would simply be a matter of adding to what they already have. They would have to ascertain whether the changes would require more fiscal and physical resources and whether sufficient resources are or can be made available. They would have to decide whether this would require a major shift in the preparation of incoming professionals and if current professionals would have to be upgraded. Even more importantly they would have to determine whether current personnel are capable of meeting or desire to meet these goals. To make the most of their programs, management would be required to refocus its decision making and establish new communication links with professionals in other fields. They would have to be willing to give up some autonomy to participate in cooperative efforts that would increase opportunities for larger segments of the population. None of this will be easy, nor will it happen overnight. Nevertheless, it must happen if the profession as a whole is to take advantage of this window of opportunity.

SPECIALIZATION

For some time there has been a trend toward specialization in the preparation of exercise-related professionals, which continues to be strong. One issue here is whether we are creating professionals with a focus that is too narrow.

Since the 1960s, professional preparation in the exercise-related professions has been marked by specialization. Immediately prior to this change, preparation centered on preparing future professionals to teach the concepts of education through the physical with a healthy dose of personal health thrown in for good measure. Once specialization took hold, physical education and health split into separate programs, each with its own curriculum.

Specialization continues today with programs developing in sport medicine/athletic training, sport management, health promotion/wellness, sport science, adult fitness, and a variety of others — each with its own curriculum and academic degree. Many, if not all, of these new specialties are supported by their own professional organizations, some of which provide various forms of certification or licensure.

The outcome of this trend is the potential for narrowing the focus in each of the specializations. That is, teaching programs could focus only on theories of teaching and transfer of information, health promotion programs might ignore the teaching of skills and fitness, athletic training programs may teach only injury prevention and treatment protocols with no attention to the athlete's personal health, and so forth.

Many believe that adding a required course here and a special topics course there can overcome this narrowing of focus. This practice, however, only deepens the split between the professional areas and does little to expand the focus of students majoring in a specific area. This is because the content is not necessarily what results in narrowing of the focus in the first place. It is the mindset of the students — a mindset that most likely comes from their major professors. The students see themselves as physical education teachers only or as athletic trainers only or as exercise scientists only.

If we are to address the challenges of the 21st century and move U. S. citizens toward a lifetime of activity, all segments of the profession must collaborate. A large part of this collaboration entails the understanding that we cannot produce professionals who have tunnel vision. These new professionals, along with those already in the profession, must see the bigger picture. They must understand that they are all physical educators and that they are all health educators. They must all promote physical activity and fitness. The physical education teacher must feel a responsibility for linking his students to community recreation and fitness programs. The athletic trainer must see her role as a health educator when working with athletes on issues such as smoking and nutrition. Recreational and fitness personnel have to see themselves as physical educators and health educators, and all of these professionals must see themselves as primary promoters of wellness. Most important, they must all see how their individual specialties are part of a whole that must work together to accomplish a common goal.

Helping future professionals do all of these things is a task for management. Decisions must be made within professional preparation programs to include material that will emphasize this concept of oneness.

Whether this is to be presented as a primary topic in one course or whether it is an objective to be accomplished in a variety of courses is a decision for program administrators to make with input from faculty and students. Administrators in these programs might have to hold special meetings with all personnel in the department to ensure that everyone is working toward the same goal.

If those responsible for teaching future professionals do not accept their role in this task, students are unlikely to adopt a philosophy that incorporates the concept that their responsibilities go beyond the boundaries of a specific specialty. They will not see the interconnectedness that is so necessary to create an environment in which people want to be, and actually are, physically active.

PROFESSIONAL DEVELOPMENT IN THE WORKPLACE

Professional development in the workplace has traditionally emphasized upgrading skills and renewing certifications and licenses. An issue here is whether this is sufficient to provide the variety of skills needed for coordinated efforts to advance the profession.

Although upgrading skills and renewing certifications and licenses are necessary aspects of continuing education, employers must see the need to go beyond these basics. As is the case in professional preparation, employers must plan time, make resources available, and encourage employees to venture into areas outside their specialties. This is no doubt carried out in some areas, but it does not take place to the extent necessary to build the links desired between the various segments of the exercise-related professions.

School teachers will not build links with community recreation and fitness programs in the public and private sectors by attending sessions at state professional conventions on new ways to incorporate fitness into their elementary program. Nor will they build these links by working toward their master's degree in administration in physical education to maintain their licensure. Athletic trainers will not become better versed at being wellness professionals by attending another seminar on the newest protocol for rehabilitating an ACL injury. Employers and professional associations need to work together to provide in-house workshops and external seminars and conventions that provide information on working together and that actually bring together the various segments of the profession to build links.

This will demand effort and time from upper management. It will not happen by waiting for someone else to do it. It will not happen as long as teachers go to one conference, coaches go to another, exercise scientists go to another, and so on. Each organization must include goals and objectives to build these links and to expand opportunities for participants through joint efforts in programming. Once established, these goals and objectives must be adequately funded and evaluated to ensure that the objectives are being met. Organizations could use the *Healthy People 2000* goals and objectives as a starting point to see where they are making similar contributions and then work to develop cooperative efforts to meet these goals and objectives. This will not be an easy task in a society where we are taught that it is every person for himself or herself in the competitive marketplace.

CERTIFICATION AND LICENSURE

There is a growing trend to require certification and licensure in a wider variety of exercise-related professions and to involve professional associations in the process of accreditation to provide more stringent quality control. An issue here is how far do we go with this trend, and will certification and licensure requiring college preparation also be required in the leisure service industry? This trend is closely associated with the first one mentioned, on common goals for exercise-related professionals. Professional preparation in exercise-related fields is closely linked to accreditation, certification, and licensure. Professional accountability is of great concern, and the exercise-related professions are no exceptions.

Major efforts are under way across the United States to upgrade professional preparation programs by involving professional organizations in setting the standards the programs and the students enrolled in these programs are to achieve. Nowhere is this more evident than in the accreditation of teacher education programs in which the National Association for Sport and Physical Education (NASPE) has developed standards used by accrediting bodies such as the National Council for the Accreditation of Teacher Education (NCATE). This same process is now under way for athletic training programs in which the Council on Accreditation of Allied Health Education Programs (CAAHEP) is establishing standards for the accreditation of programs whose graduates will ultimately be certified by the National Athletic Trainers Association Board of Certification (NATABOC).

Teacher education programs that want to maintain their accreditation are having to take long, hard looks at their programs to determine whether they can meet the new standards formulated by NASPE. Because these standards require students to exhibit specific skills and knowledge, administrators must identify potential deficiencies and decide what additional course content is needed to overcome these deficiencies. It must also be determined whether additional practicum hours are needed, whether adequate numbers of master teachers are available for practicum assignments, and how students will be supervised during these practicums. All of this must be considered in light of a stable or decreasing demand for physical education teachers and whether fewer enrollees in teacher preparation programs warrant greater expenditures to meet the new standards. Some programs have decided the increased expense is not warranted and have dropped programs.

Virtually the same situation exists in athletic training programs. Whereas NATABOC currently accepts candidates for certification from both internship-type training programs and curricular programs, beginning in 2004 it will accept candidates only from curricular programs. Further those curricular programs must meet standards from and be accredited by CAAHEP. (NATABOC may require standards in addition to those imposed by CAAHEP.) Institutions that have had successful curricular or internship programs but are not accredited must now decide whether they have resources available to meet the accreditation standards. Likely, many will realize that they will not have the necessary resources and will drop their athletic training programs, thereby allowing available resources to be concentrated on other programs.

Accreditation of programs that produce graduates who are certifiable or licensable is a method of quality control. Quality control is certainly an issue in the exercise-related professions and demands the support of all of those in the profession. Quality control, however, seems to be at its highest in fields in which the professionals are already better prepared — those that require a college degree. Teachers, athletic trainers, physical therapists, and most recreational specialists not only must graduate from an accredited program but also must pass a national or state certification or licensure exam. This is not the case for coaches, fitness instructors, and most of the personnel who make up the rapidly growing leisure–services industry.

Certifications are available for these professionals. Although some professions highly recommend the certifications, they are not required. Many coaches in school and recreational settings have no training in coaching techniques, much less in physiology and psychology. Some areas do require certifications for recreational coaches but, because most recreational-level coaches are volunteers and budgets are limited, the certification is minimal at best. With higher interest in sport participation nationwide in general and increased interest from females and older adults in particular, this situation is likely to get worse before it gets better.

If that situation is not bad enough, the personal trainer or aerobic dance instructor working with the growing number of participants in the leisure-services industry may have nothing more than a high school education. This does not mean that these individuals cannot be skilled at what they do. Many are, and some even are certified by one of the many fitness-certifying bodies available across the United States. Some of these certifying bodies, such as the American College of Sports Medicine (ACSM), do require a college degree, or at least completion of college-level courses. Nevertheless, no mechanism is available that mandates these certifications to ensure any standard of quality control. Other certifying bodies require nothing more than a warm body and a certification fee. The only control available is the pressure of the marketplace. If enough consumers are not satisfied due to the quality of service and care they are receiving, the business might not survive.

An issue here is whether the pressure of the marketplace is sufficient to provide the level of quality control necessary to protect the consumer and to advance the message of the importance of physical activity in a way that will keep participants involved and not turned off. Lacking that, what must be done to provide appropriate quality control? In a free-market society, that answer is not easy. Professionals in the exercise-related fields must help educate the public concerning quality control and hope for public pressure to create a demand for higher standards and certifications.

If this should come about, numerous management questions will be raised, for which answers must be found. These will start at the professional preparation level, at which programs must do a better job of preparing graduates to function in the private sector. Running a business and dealing with a paying customer require skills not obtained in a typical fitness/wellness undergraduate program. Management decisions would certainly have to be made within the leisure-services industry as well. Providing a program conducted by uncertified, minimally trained employees cannot be offered at the same cost as a program requiring certified, college graduates. Of course, improved programs reaching customers with more diverse needs could be offered. These programming concerns are directly related to several issues that follow.

PRIVATIZATION OF LEISURE-PURSUIT OPPORTUNITIES

Privatization of leisure-pursuit

There is a trend toward the privatization of leisure-pursuit opportunities, resulting in a trend in which opportunities are limited to only those who can afford them. The issue here is whether these trends will make it impossible for the profession to ever reach its goal of lifelong participation for everyone.

The leisure–service industry is by and large a private industry. "Private" does not necessarily mean "private club" with exclusive membership, even though that is certainly part of the leisure-service industry. "Private" refers to privately owned rather than publicly operated. Bowling alleys, golf complexes, fitness centers, ski resorts, ice and roller skating rinks, athletic centers, outdoor adventure businesses, and the like are all privately owned. Yes, some golf courses and ice rinks are found within state and county parks. For the most part, though, these exist in the private sector. Customers must pay to avail themselves of the opportunities for activity that these businesses offer. The costs of some of these are significant, especially golf courses and ski resorts.

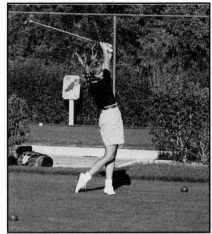

Physical activity that is fun encourages young people to become more active.

In addition to the cost of paying for the activity itself, participants must pay for the equipment used in these activities. This brings them into contact with another part of the leisure service industry — merchandising. Even when people are participating in a publicly sponsored activity, they most likely have spent a significant sum of money to purchase the needed equipment. The same is true when providing one's own opportunities, such as boating, camping, and even jogging and walking.

This private industry provides the adult population with a significant portion of its activity opportunities — that is, if you are an adult with the means to pay for the opportunity. The segment of our society that lives on a limited and often fixed income with little, if any, discretionary resources cannot and does not make use of these opportunities. In this group — the economically deprived and many elderly citizens — hypokinetic diseases wreak the greatest havoc.

From a management perspective, can we expect private industry to adjust its programming and what it charges for programs to allow individuals with limited economic resources to take advantage of these opportunities? The answer is, "probably not." Can we expect some redistribution of wealth that would provide "activity welfare" to the economically deprived? The atmosphere for "giveaways" over the last decade has not been good and is not likely to be any better in the future. About the only way to deal with this issue is to overcome the next trend.

AGE-RANGE OF PARTICIPATION

In a long-term trend, public sponsored programs have been primarily for children, youths, and young adults. The issue here is whether public programs can expand sufficiently to provide activities over the entire age range and, even if they can, whether the segments of society who need these opportunities can be convinced to participate in them.

Pay-to-play

Municipal and county recreational programs make up the largest portion of our public-activity opportunities. State and federal programs, usually in the public park system, add some programs. Many of these, however, are accessible only by paying a fee, so they are not much different from those in the private sector. As a matter of fact, one trend in the public sector is *pay-to-play* in which participants are charged to play in a variety of sport-oriented activities. Although minimal registration fees have been a part of public recreation for some time, pay-to-play goes beyond that. Pay-to-play is designed to more fully support the activity, whereas registration fees were instituted to collect small amounts of revenue to offset the cost of programs.

Recreation programs have had to resort to these measures to fund their programs in a time when the public in general is not willing to pay more and more taxes to support public programs of any type. If these programs must charge fees to provide programs to a limited age group, how can they be expected to offer programs to a wider age range without increasing fees even more? Working with preschoolers and older adults requires a lower participant-to-instructor ratio. Working with each of these groups also requires personnel who are specially trained to work with them. Both of these conditions increase the costs of the programs. And if higher costs result in higher fees, the public sector will not be much different from the private sector. We should note that pay-to-play policies have been challenged in the courts and supported by the courts as long as provisions are made to exempt the economically deprived from paying the fees.

Public recreation can certainly expand to meet the needs of participants over a wider age range. Administrators can devise programs to meet a variety of needs. Personnel can be trained to work with individuals of any age. As a society, though, are we willing to let ourselves be taxed to provide for additional personnel, programs, and facilities? As a profession, are we willing to make the hard sell to the public — to convince people of the benefits to be gained from a lifetime of physical activity?

Are those of us in a position to help take some of the burden off public recreation willing to do so? Can schools become sites of public activity wherein students and parents come to participate together on week nights and weekends in programs offered by physical education teachers who now become public recreators? Talk about a programming change, a management marvel! What a great opportunity for teachers to see skills they taught earlier put into action. What a great opportunity to see families play together and work toward building a lifetime fitness program together. A pipe dream? Maybe.

Of course, even programs such as this would have their cost. We could not expect a teacher to teach all day and then work in the evenings and on weekends (unless he or she is a coach). Some system of staggered schedules would have to be initiated, and full-time recreators would have to be involved in the programs. But at least facilities would be duplicated less often and management expertise would be available from teachers, coaches, and principals. Teachers could even use material from the life-span development courses they are now required to take.

SCHOOL PROGRAMS

There is a growing public perception that school programs in both physical education and athletics are no longer meeting their objectives. Physical education programs are often seen as ineffective, and varsity athletic programs as exclusionary. Regardless of the area of specialty in exercise-related professions, we are no doubt familiar with these opinions. We can conjure up visions of roll-the-ball-out physical education classes with teachers asleep in the bleachers and athletic teams on which only the chosen few ever get to play. We can see youngsters who will grow up to be adults who have nothing but negative memories about always being chosen last in the physical education class or never making the B–team, much less the varsity team. Are these accurate pictures of physical education and athletics? In far too many situations the answer is "yes." In more and more situations, though, this is not the case.

Exclusionary (sports program)

Physical education programs across the country are adopting the new content standards from the National Association for Sport and Physical Education that indicate a high-quality program. In some cases these standards are simply a means of validating the programs already in place. For others the standards have triggered significant changes that required lengthy planning sessions resulting in immediate change for some and gradual change for others — change that is still in process for many.

Many youngsters get their only opportunity to experience organized physical activity in the physical education class. The 1996 Surgeon General's Report on *Physical Activity and Health* notes that this is minimal time for many; only 19% of students attending physical education classes daily indicated that they were participating actively for more than 20 minutes. No doubt time is a major factor in physical education — too little for each class, too seldom throughout the year, and not far enough into the school grades. Many elementary students are in physical education classes only once or twice a week; many middle school students meet in physical education classes every day for only one of the 9-week periods during the year; and many high school students complete only a 1-unit requirement in the ninth grade.

From a management perspective, little can be done to increase the time allotted. The physical educator must be able to create an atmosphere that is most conducive to learning — an atmosphere in which the students look forward to participating in the planned activities. Some controversy is voiced as to whether the limited time available should be spent in movement and skills or whether more time should be given to fitness development. In some cases, edicts from state departments or school district coordinators will determine the primary focus. In others individual teachers or departments will decide. Whatever the case, those who are presenting the programs must remember that they can have a major influence on whether a child chooses to be active throughout life or not.

A trend strongly related to inactivity must be mentioned at this point. When physical education teachers are attempting to interest their students in physical activity, they must always be aware that they are competing against a powerful foe. That foe is technology. Today's technology encourages inactivity. Labor-saving devices are intended to be nonlabor-intensive. At the same time, they are supposed to allow more leisure time. But then along comes another form of technology to use during leisure time.

Computers and computer games mesmerize young users — and older users as well. The player can defend New York City against Godzilla, drive the world's most famous race courses, or play the most challenging golf courses on the professional golf tour without ever leaving home. So when teachers are thinking about how stimulating they have to make their fitness class, they had better set their stimulator high if they expect their influence to match or exceed the computer that is beckoning at home.

Success, or lack thereof, in varsity sports can also have a major influence in whether a person chooses to be active throughout life. Those of us who have had positive experiences in sport see it as beneficial and seek to continue participation as long as possible at some level. Those who have had negative experiences might not even be active spectators, much less active participants. Since its inception, the U. S. sports system has been one of gradual exclusion. The early levels feature many teams with few rules, and everyone is encouraged to play and have fun. As we get older, the teams become fewer, the rules become more important, and the game becomes more serious. We are dejected when we try out for the team and do not make it, or disgusted when we do make it but never get to play. Many do not try out at all because they think they have no chance to make the team. By the time we are adults, we have lost interest in participating in sports altogether.

This does not present an attractive picture of sports. Yet we are crazy about sports in this society, and in much of the world the feeling is the same. We like to connect with the athlete's success. We might even want to "be like Michael," even though we know we never will. The system that leads us to this point has little chance of being anything but exclusionary. Schools do as much as they possibly can to field junior varsity,

B-teams, and varsity teams for males and females alike. We cannot expect them to field "almost B-teams." We can, however, expect intramural programs, after-school programs, and weekend programs offered exclusively by the school or in conjunction with recreation departments. We can expect sport club systems to provide opportunities not only for school-aged children and youth but for adults as well.

This raises additional questions about programming, personnel, and funding, and these questions can be answered. The solutions ultimately have to involve many different players. Ultimately, though, those in the exercise-related professions have to ask the questions and take the initial actions to bring about these types of programs. If programs of this nature are not instituted, we will miss an opportunity to positively effect people's attitudes about lifelong physical activity.

EQUITY IN SPORT

Sport has long been male-dominated. In the area of participation, this has resulted in large part to myths about the female's capability to withstand physical stress. Scientific study and actual experience have long showed this myth to be just that — a myth. Nevertheless, old beliefs die hard, especially when supported by prejudices and stereotypes of what is feminine and what is not. For many years, being physically active was not seen as a feminine characteristic and, worse yet, females who were active were seen as not being female at all. A male-dominated medical profession often warned about damage to a woman's ability to bear children if she were to participate in strenuous exercise. For the most part, we are beyond those beliefs, and change is occurring, though at a slow pace.

Equity in sport

The 1972 Educational Amendments to the Civil Rights Act of 1964 have resulted in significant gains in opportunities for females in sport. This law stipulates that no educational program receiving federal funds can discriminate against anyone based on sex, and Title IX of the act applies this stipulation to the area of sport (and physical education). This law, however, did not eliminate discrimination against females in sport. Although the law does give them a remedy when discrimination occurs, they still have to fight the battle. If discrimination is present and no one complains, the discrimination persists.[1]

Even though gains in sport have resulted from Title IX, work remains to be done. Shortages of coaches and funds make it difficult to offer needed programs. Often, where honest efforts are being made to improve opportunities for females, programs might have to be reduced for males because of the balancing act that is necessary when resources are limited. Also, the quality of coaching and programming may be less than desired

Title IX

in programs for males and females because of lack of funds. Title IX was not intended to decrease opportunities for males or to decrease the quality of programs offered.

If we believe that participation in sport is a valid experience in our educational programs — and it is fairly obvious that we do — we should be willing to support these programs. If we do not, as a profession and as individuals, programming will continue to be less than it could be and we will have missed another opportunity to establish a positive attitude toward physical activity in a large segment of our society.

Obviously, equity in sport goes beyond the issue of numbers of female teams versus male teams. It also goes to opportunity to participate based on race and age. Even though we probably do not intentionally discriminate because of age, we do have far more programs for youths than we do for the elderly, particularly in the public sector. Even though discrimination against race is more likely to be intentional, unintentional discrimination has the same effect. When more funds are spent for new recreational facilities in locations that are more likely to be used by people from predominantly white neighborhoods and little or no money is spent in predominantly minority neighborhoods, we have discriminated.

Selective programming

Discrimination is often the result of lack of planning that results in selective programming as well as poorly placed recreational facilities. Selective programming is that type of programming that attracts a certain clientele. This is not because one racial group or the other does not have the ability to perform a given activity but because they have no experience in, and therefore no interest in, that activity. From a management perspective, this puts the onus on the administration to be familiar with the demographics of the area and plan programs and place facilities that will attract participants of all ages and races.

Last but not least is the issue of equity in employment in sport. This issue is constantly in the sporting news. Will a black be hired for this job, or will a female be hired for that job, or will this person get this job because she is a black female? Of course, these are the high-profile jobs — the ones that make the news. But the same questions are being asked every day in all sporting venues. And the answers continue to be the same: "Probably not." In the case of females, even when they are hired, will they get the same salary as their male counterparts? Again, the answer is: "Probably not." What can be done about this? Individuals should persist and make use of equal opportunity of employment and equal pay laws when they believe they have been discriminated against. As a profession, we can certainly support efforts to combat discrimination through joint efforts and support equal opportunity through our personal actions.

What management perspective is involved here? Other than the obvious one of avoiding discrimination in who we hire and what we do to attract professionals of all races is a programming note that we probably overlook more than we should. Participants, especially younger participants, look to their coaches, teachers, recreators, athletic trainers, and fitness leaders as role models. If young women do not see a female in these positions, and if young Black males or young Hispanic males or young Asian males never see a Black, or Hispanic, or Asian male leader in these positions, what influence can we expect the activity to have on them in the long term? Even if it is a positive experience in general, it will not be as positive as it could have been and we shall have failed to interest another group in lifelong physical activity.

NOTES

1. N. J. Dougherty et al. (1994). *Sport, Physical Activity, and the Law*. Champaign, IL: Human Kinetics.

RESOURCES

Dougherty, N. J., et al. (1994). *Sport, Physical Activity, and the Law*. Champaign, IL: Human Kinetics Publishers.

Educational Amendment Act of 1972 (P. L. 92–318, 86 Stat. 373), 20 U.S.C. 1681 (a)(1).

Lumpkin, A. (1998). *Physical Education and Sport, A Contemporary Introduction*, 4th ed. Boston: WCB/McGraw-Hill.

Siedentop, D. (1998). *Introduction to Physical Education, Fitness, and Sport*, 3d ed. Mountain View, CA: Mayfield Publishing.

U. S. Public Health Service. (1991). *Healthy People 2000: National Health Promotion and Disease Objectives* (DHHS Publication No. [PHS] 91–50212). Washington, DC:

U. S. Government Printing Office.U. S. Department of Health and Human Services. (1996). *Physical Activity and Health: A Report of the Surgeon General*. Atlanta: U. S. Department of Health and Human Services, Centers for Disease Control and Prevention, National Center for Chronic Disease Prevention and Health Promotion.

Wuest, D. A., & C. A. Bucher (1995). *Foundations of Physical Education and Sport*, 12th ed. St. Louis: Mosby-Yearbook.

Principles and Concepts of Organization

OBJECTIVES

After studying this chapter, you should be able to:

1. Explain the nature of the term *organization* and its importance to the success of a program.
2. Identify and discuss the seven principles of the organizational process.
3. Define and explain the following organizational concepts:
   a. scope of responsibility
   b. delegation of responsibility and authority
   c. doctrine of unity

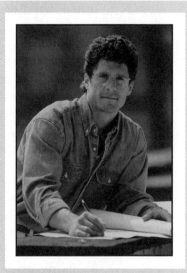

Organization

O*rganization* is both a process and a product. As a *process*, organization means developing a systematic plan to accomplish the program and institutional goals. As a *product*, organization is the framework, the institutional structure that results from the process of organizational planning. The main goal of the organizational process and establishment of an organizational framework is to maximize the effectiveness of available resources. The specific logistics of the organizational process are presented in Chapter 4.

Principles

Principles are guidelines that, when utilized, improve the probability of success. Every discipline has principles that govern critical processes. For example, accountants recognize and utilize sound principles of accounting to correctly and efficiently complete their work. Students of grammar use specific principles to diagram and analyze sentence structure. In the same manner, the study of organization and administration begins with sound principles of administration (see Chapter 5) and organization. These are explored in the remainder of this chapter.

A MEANS TO AN END

Organization is viewed as a means to an end rather than an end in itself. In the world of professional sports, certain franchises are recognized as "great organizations," largely due to their consistent success in their respective sports. This might lead to the conclusion that the purpose of devoting time and effort to developing of an effective organizational plan is to produce an end product (the organization) worthy of recognition. Actually, development of an effective organizational plan is simply a way to achieve the goals — the success for which the organization is striving. Great professional sports organizations are recognized for their "greatness" because of numerous championships and continued financial success, not because of a beautiful, well-conceived organizational plan that hangs in the office of the organization's CEO.

In much the same way that the true beauty of a super highway lies in its ability to enable travelers to get to their desired destination and not in the steel and concrete of the highway itself, the beauty of an effective organizational plan lies in its ability to facilitate the organization's attaining its desired goals. For example, an effectively organized college athletics program or corporate fitness program is more likely to reap the rewards of success than a program that lacks clear organizational direction.

SCOPE OF RESPONSIBILITY

Scope of responsibility

An effective organizational plan reflects a clear understanding of the "scope of responsibility" concept. Scope of responsibility refers to the breadth or extent of one's responsibility within an organization. For example, a head athletic trainer's *scope of responsibility* is larger than that of an assistant athletic trainer. The former is responsible for all aspects of, and all personnel within, the athletic training program, whereas an assistant athletic trainer has a lesser *scope of responsibility*, involving only selected program components and personnel.

When developing an organizational plan, the organizers must recognize and plan for an appropriate scope of responsibility for each member of the organization. If an employee is given a scope of responsibility that is too large or too small, the result can be disastrous, for the individual and the organization alike.

For example, a young, inexperienced Director of Intramurals who is given responsibility for all intramural sports activities, all campus recreation activities, *and* the supervision of all campus physical education and recreational facilities may not be able to effectively carry out all of her responsibilities. This may represent an environmental/circumstantial job performance problem (see Chapter 9). On the other hand, an experienced physical education instructor who is given little administrative responsibility may feel underutilized, underappreciated, and even bored, resulting in a motivation/incentive performance problem (see Chapter 9). Therefore, decisions concerning appropriate scope of responsibility should be made prior to the development of, and reflected within the organizational plan.

DELEGATION OF RESPONSIBILITY AND AUTHORITY

An effective organizational plan should reflect clear understanding of the "delegation of responsibility and authority" concept. As discussed in Chapters 5 and 6, an effective administrator is one who has learned to delegate appropriate responsibilities to key members throughout the organization. Delegation allows employees with specific experience, talents, or interests to assume specific responsibilities, and, thus, more effectively utilize the strengths of organizational personnel. For example, an assistant coach with extensive experience and interest in designing and implementing physical conditioning programs may be delegated the responsibility for the off-season physical conditioning program. This assignment should be formally reflected in the Athletics Department's organizational plan.

Delegation of responsibility and authority

Although the delegation of appropriate responsibilities is a cornerstone of successful organizations, an effective administrator understands that the delegation of responsibility is not enough. Along with the responsibility, appropriate authority to carry out the responsibility must be delegated. In the above example, assigning responsibility for off-season conditioning to an assistant coach will be of little value if he is not also given the authority to run the program (to establish conditioning program policies, to discipline athletes who violate conditioning program policies, and so on). Delegated responsibilities and authority go hand-in-hand and should be clearly reflected in the organizational plan.

LINES OF FORMAL COMMUNICATION

An effective organizational plan clearly establishes the appropriate lines of formal communication. Chapter 8 presents a detailed explanation of organizational communication. As noted there, formal communication takes place along established organizational communication lines. For example, if an exercise specialist in a cardiac rehabilitation program has a concern about her work schedule, her first contact should be with her immediate supervisor. In a large program, she may work directly under the supervision of a Head Exercise Specialist; in a small program, she may report directly to the Program Director. The organizational plan should clearly delineate appropriate lines of communication that all organizational personnel are to utilize.

DOCTRINE OF UNITY

Doctrine of unity   *An effective organizational plan reflects clear understanding of the "doctrine of unity."* In any type of organization, functions of a similar nature and with similar goals and objectives should be grouped into administrative units. This is known as the doctrine of unity. For example, a college or university Physical Education Department might have three major functions:

1. The department might have a major program in physical education teacher preparation.

2. The department might have a degree program in athletic training.

3. The department might offer a wide variety of general education physical activity courses (tennis, golf, swimming, racquetball, and so on).

Therefore, these functional areas (physical education teacher preparation, athletic training, and physical activity services) should be placed in separate administrative units for easier and more effective administration. The department's organizational plan should clearly illustrate these three distinct administrative units.

COORDINATION AND COOPERATION

An effective organizational plan should reflect clear understanding of the importance of coordination and cooperation among administrative units within the organization. Organizations with multiple administrative units must be designed to encourage and facilitate coordination and cooperation among these units. The larger and more diverse the organization, the more critical this principle becomes. For example, a large Department of Athletics may contain numerous sports (both male and female), a sports medicine or athletic training program, a sports information and marketing program, an athlete recruiting program, a financial program, and an education and eligibility compliance program, each under the direct supervision of an assistant director of athletics. Even though each of these programs is designed to fulfill unique goals and objectives of the total athletic program, all of their efforts should be undertaken in full coordination and cooperation with all the other facets of the athletics program.

Without planned coordination, otherwise-effective sports medicine services, for example, might disintegrate into chaos and confusion if athletes from five different sports report to the training room at the same time requesting taping and other treatment. Conversely, the thoughtful coordination of practice schedules and cooperation of athletic trainers, coaches, and athletes can result in a smooth, effective day-to-day working relationship. Numerous other examples could be cited from any exercise-related organization. The main point is that coordination and cooperation must be considered in the development of, and reflected in, the organizational plan.

A SPECIFIC ORGANIZATIONAL PLAN

An organizational plan is designed to meet the specific needs of the organization for which it is developed. Last, but certainly not of least significance, is the caveat that each and every organization and program is unique, and, therefore, each and every organizational plan should be custom-designed to reflect the specific nature of the organization or program. No plan should be cloned from another existing organization — regardless of how similar it may be — or from some textbook (this one included).

RESOURCES

Arburgey, T. L. (1993). Resetting the clock: The dynamics of organizational change and failure. *Administrative Science Quarterly*, March: 51–73.

Draft, R. L. (1992). *Organizational Theory and Design*, 4th ed. St. Paul, MN: West Publishing.

Johns, G. (1988). *Organizational Behavior: Understanding Life at Work*, 2d. ed. Glenview, IL: Scott, Foresman.

Robbins, S. (1990). *Organization Theory: Structure, Design, and Applications*. Englewood Cliffs, NJ: Prentice-Hall.

Developing An Effective Organizational Plan

OBJECTIVES

After studying this chapter, you should be able to:

1. Explain the purposes of an effective organizational plan.

2. Interpret simple line-staff and circular organizational plans.

3. Identify, in proper sequence, the seven steps involved in developing an effective organizational plan.

4. Discuss and follow the process of developing an effective organizational plan.

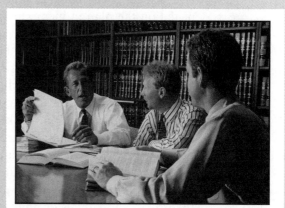

As discussed in Chapter 3, an organizational plan is a written framework that represents the responsibility, authority, and communication relationships within an organization. More specifically, an organizational plan is a tool that may be used to (a) provide a conceptual overview of an organization, (b) enhance understanding of the administrative structure of the organization, and (c) clarify specific lines of authority and communication among the various components of an organization.

Organizational plan

UNDERSTANDING ORGANIZATIONAL PLANS

The final organizational principle in Chapter 3 pointed out that no two organizational plans are alike, nor should they be. From a broad perspective, however, two widely used organizational plans are the line-staff plan and the circular plan.

Line-Staff Plan

Line-staff plan

The most common form of organizational plan is known as a *line-staff plan* because solid lines (——) and broken lines (- - - -) are used to illustrate relationships among the various administrative units and persons represented in the plan. Administrative units and personnel are also depicted on the plan in hierarchical order. The higher one's position on the chart, the greater is his or her responsibility and authority.

Lines of responsibility

In a line-staff plan, vertical lines indicate formal lines of responsibility. Individuals or units are responsible for functions that are below them and connected to them either directly or indirectly by solid vertical lines. Solid horizontal lines connect individuals or units of comparable authority or status in the organization. Broken lines generally represent lines of informal (advisory) communication between individuals or units that are not connected by lines of formal authority or communication. Broken lines also may be used to depict relationships between (a) staff positions (such as an administrative assistant) and individuals or units of authority, and (b) affiliate individuals or units (such as the team physician) and individuals or units of authority. A simple line-staff plan is shown in Figure 4.1.

*Status
Informal
communication*

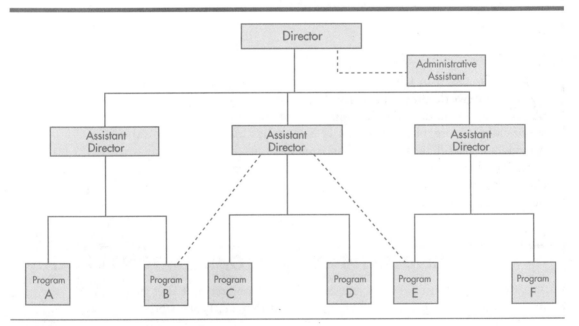

FIGURE 4.1   *Simple Line-Staff Plan*

Circular Plan

A *circular organizational plan* utilizes a series of concentric circles to repre-   *Circular plan*
sent responsibility, authority, and communication relationships. Individuals
and units of greater authority reside at or along the inner circles, and individuals or units of lesser authority are positioned on outer circles. Individuals or units are located along the same circle when they are of comparable
authority and organizational status. As with the line-staff design, lines of
formal authority and communication are represented by solid, connecting
lines, whereas broken lines represent staff relationships and informal lines
of communication. A simple circular plan is shown in Figure 4.2.

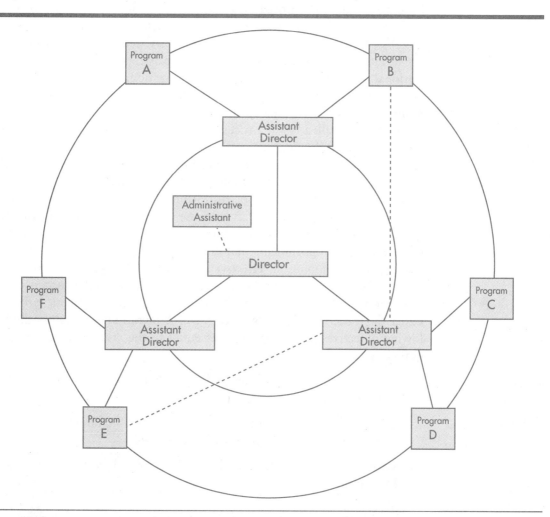

FIGURE 4.2 *Simple Circular Plan*

Other Plans

A wide variety of other organizational designs is available. Most of these are unique designs reflecting the specific configuration of the organizations they represent. Therefore, the remainder of this chapter will utilize the common line-staff organizational concept.

THE PROCESS OF DEVELOPING AN ORGANIZATIONAL PLAN

Every organization and every program within an organization should have a formal, written organizational plan. Without a formal plan, lines of authority and communication are often unclear and difficult, if not impossible, to understand. The typical result is that each person within the organization or program develops his or her own perception of the organizational structure. Therefore, a clear organizational plan is essential if the delegation of responsibilities and authority and appropriate lines of communication are to be clearly understood. An administrator, therefore, must become skilled in the process of developing an organizational plan, set forth in the following steps.

1. *Establish and recognize organizational goals and objectives*. The importance of organizational goals and objectives is discussed in detail in Chapter 5. Every successful organization and program has established specific goals that define the very purpose of the organization or program. To attain these goals, numerous short-term and long-term objectives identify specific accomplishments that must be realized in the process. The initial step in developing an effective organizational plan is to establish a "master list" of goals and objectives that are critical to the success of the organization or program. For example, a high school athletic program under the leadership of a new Director of Athletics might identify the following objectives as among those essential to the attainment of the programs goals:

- Within 3 years, the program will field two new girls' teams and two new boys' teams.

- In each of the first 3 years of the program, a minimum of two new community financial sponsors will be secured.

- Membership in the school's athletics booster club will be increased by 25% in the first year.

2. *Identify the specific tasks and functions necessary for meeting stated goals and objectives*. As discussed in Chapter 5, goals and objectives

are of little value unless strategies are developed for reaching them. Therefore, every goal, short-term objective, and long-term objective should be supported by a list of tasks and functions (strategies) that will be employed to meet the stated goals and objectives.

For example, a hospital-based cardiac rehabilitation program may have as one of its primary goals to maintain a certain level of enrollment for services to remain cost-effective. Therefore, objectives and strategies for achieving this goal must be developed. It may be determined that some of the critical "enrollment maintenance" strategies are to include (a) increasing the variety of rehabilitation activities available, (b) expanding the number of hours per day during which the program will be available, (c) adding client-education sessions to the current selection of client activities, and (d) creating a plan for personally contacting all cardiologists and internists in the surrounding five-county area to solicit their support of the program.

Every organizational goal will have numerous short-term and long-term objectives, and every objective will have strategies that must be employed if the objectives are to be met and the goals accomplished. Identifying these strategies is crucial to the process of developing the organizational plan.

3. *Group organizational objectives according to the similarity of their related tasks and functions.* Once objectives and related strategies have been identified, objectives should be grouped according to the similarity of their related strategies. For example, when developing an intramural sports program, objectives with strategies relating to facility management should be grouped together, as should those dealing with team recruitment and league formation. Simply stated, place activities together that "go together" (see doctrine of unity, Chapter 3).

4. *Place the grouped objectives into appropriate administrative units (departments).* Grouping objectives with related strategies enables them to be placed in appropriate administrative units. For example, a college or university groups similar academic disciplines into logical administrative units (School of Nursing, Division of Mathematics and Computer Science, Department of Physical Education and Exercise Sciences). In turn, the Department of Physical Education and Exercise Sciences may be composed of four distinct functional units (Physical Education Teacher Education program, Exercise Science program, Athletic Training Education program, and Physical Activity Service program). Because of their similar goals, objectives, and strategies, these four programs become individual administrative units.

Administrative units

When establishing these units, the concept of *scope of responsibility* must be carefully considered to avoid creating administrative units so large that effective administration and supervision of their activities would be impractical. Therefore, creating two or more smaller sub-units within some administrative units may be a consideration. Within this step actual creation of the written organizational plan begins to take shape.

5. *Utilizing the administrative units established in the previous step, prepare a model plan.* Now you are ready to put your model organizational plan on paper. Utilizing the guidelines for line-staff planning, an organizational plan can be designed to accurately represent the administrative structure that has been created. When completed, anyone with knowledge of the line-staff concept should be able to look at the finished plan and quickly and easily understand (a) the specific administrative structure of the organization, and (b) the specific lines of authority and communication within the organization.

6. *Implement the proposed organizational plan.* The plan is simply a means to accomplish the goals of the organization, so it must be utilized. It has been suggested that there is no such thing as a good idea that will not work. Similarly, there is no such thing as a good organizational plan that will not work. The key is to put the plan into action.

For example, an organizational plan for an athletic training program may have separate administrative units for Men's Sports and Women's Sports and may include an affiliate relationship with a Medical Team. On paper, these designations are of little value. Only when a Head Athletic Trainer for Men's Sports, a Head Athletic Trainer for Women's Sports, and a team of affiliate medical specialists are actually in place and functioning can the plan "come to life."

7. *Periodically evaluate the organizational plan and modify it as deemed necessary for optimal effectiveness.* With few exceptions, organizational plans look great on paper. In truth, most plans require continuous modification and fine-tuning in order to remain effective. Therefore, periodic evaluation is crucial to the continuing success of any organizational plan.

Figures 4.3–4.11 contain sample organizational plans for various exercise-related organizations and programs.

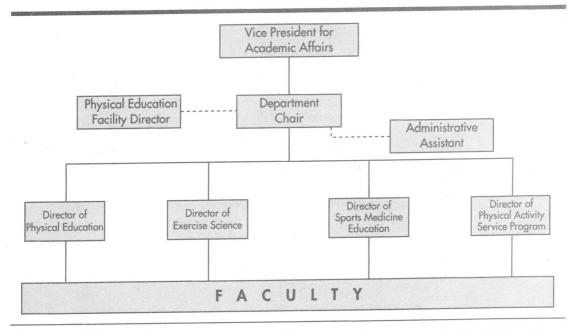

FIGURE 4.3 *Sample Organizational Plan: College/University Department of Physical Education and Exercise Science*

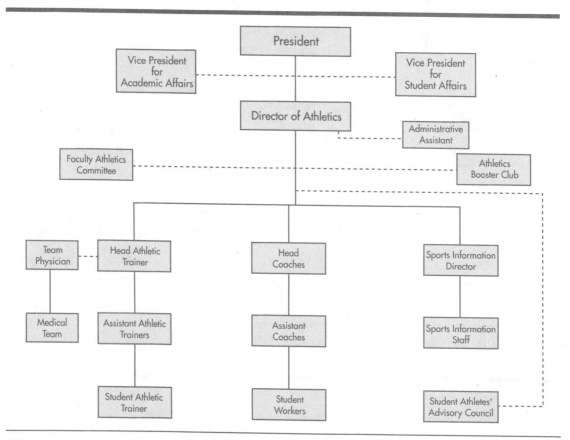

FIGURE 4.4 *Sample Organizational Plan: Small-College Department of Athletics*

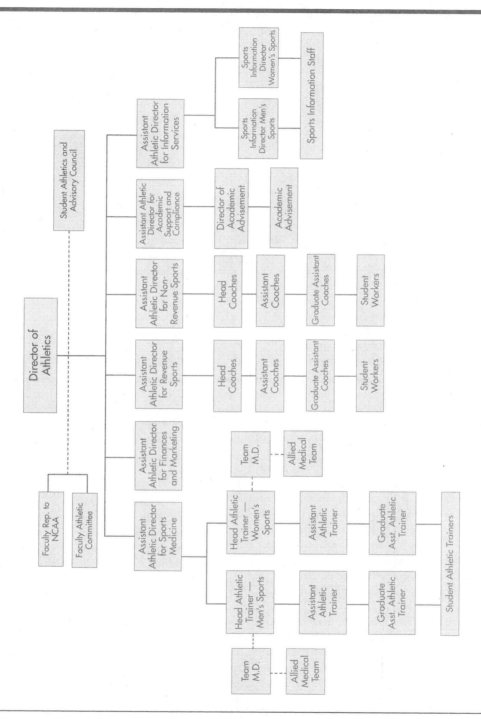

FIGURE 4.5 *Sample Organizational Plan: Large-University Department of Athletics*

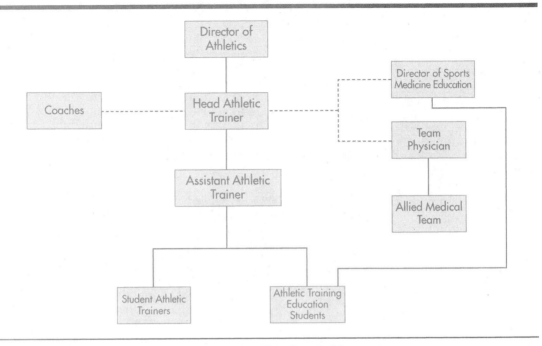

FIGURE 4.6   *Sample Organizational Plan: Small-College Athletic Training Program*

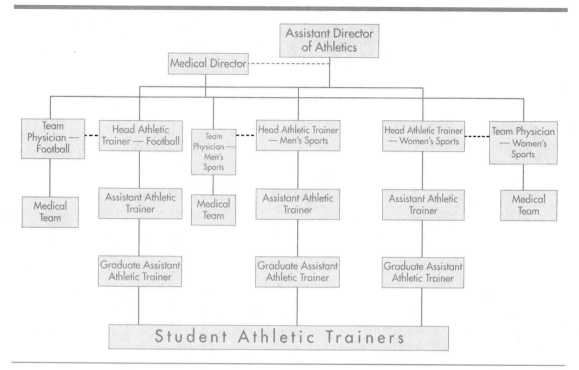

FIGURE 4.7 *Sample Organizational Chart: Large-University Athletic Training Program*

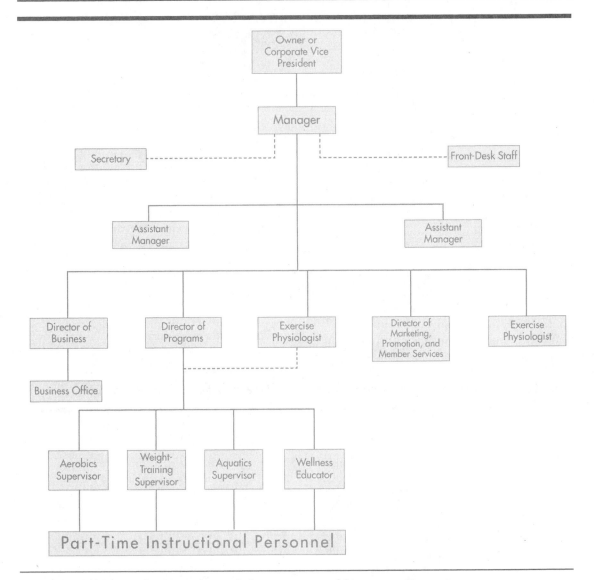

FIGURE 4.8 *Sample Organizational Plan: Commercial/Corporate Fitness Program*

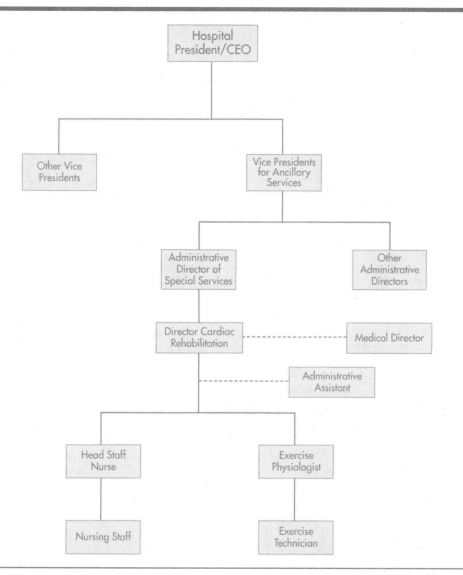

FIGURE 4.9 *Sample Organizational Plan: Cardiac Rehabilitation Program*

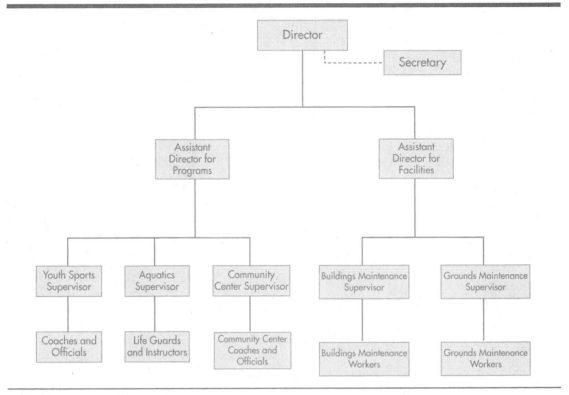

FIGURE 4.10 *Sample Organizational Chart: Parks and Recreation Department*

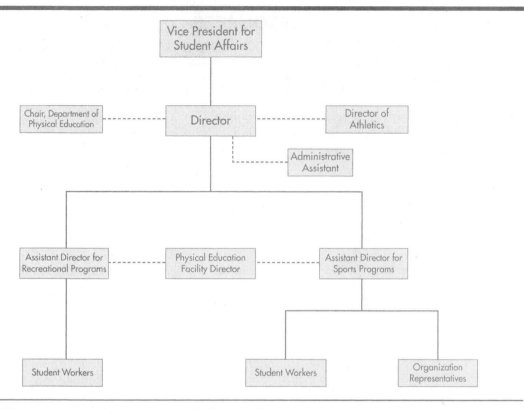

FIGURE 4.11   *Sample Organizational Chart: College/University Intramural Activities Program*

RESOURCES

Draft, R. L. (1992). *Organizational Theory and Design*, 4th ed. St. Paul, MN: West Publishing.

McCann, J. E. (1991). Design principles for an innovating company. *Academy of Management Executive*, 5:76–93.

Mintzberg, H. (1979). *The Structuring of Organizations*. Englewood Cliffs, NJ: Prentice–Hall.

Slack, T. and C. R. Hinings. (1987). Planning and organizational change: A conceptual framework for the analysis of amateur sport organizations. *Canadian Journal of Sport Sciences*, 12:185–193.

5

Principles and Concepts of Administration

OBJECTIVES

After studying this chapter, you should be able to:

1. Explain the nature of the term *administration* and its importance to the success of a program or organization.

2. Identify and discuss the six principles of effective administration.

3. Define and explain the concept of outcome-based administration.

4. Identify the five components of an effective performance-based objective.

5. Write effective outcome-based performance-based objectives.

6. Utilize performance-based objectives effectively in the process of administration.

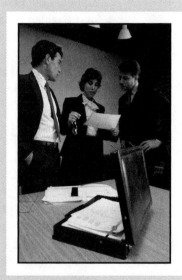

Administration

A*dministration* is the process of guiding, leading, and coordinating the efforts of a group of individual people or segments within an organization toward the attainment of organizational (program and institutional) goals. As discussed earlier with the organizational process, administration is simply a means to an end — that end being the common goals of the organization. For a high school physical education program, a common goal may be to graduate students who have an appreciation for physical activity, whereas an athletic training program may have a goal of developing an effective injury-prevention program for all sports. The role of administration, therefore, is to provide guidance, leadership, and coordination of the efforts of the physical education or athletic training staff toward the realization of these goals.

PRINCIPLES OF ADMINISTRATION

As previously stated, principles are guidelines that, if followed, enhance the probability of success. Administration is more likely to be effective when the following fundamental principles of the administrative process are utilized.

Organizational philosophy

Organizational goals

1. *Administrative activities are consistent with organizational philosophy and directed toward attainment of organizational goals (desired outcomes).* Every organization and every program reflects the philosophy upon which it is founded. One athletics program may be driven by the philosophy that success is measured in wins and championships. Another program may measure success in financial terms, striving to become self-supporting through revenues the program generates. Likewise, the philosophy behind one company's corporate wellness program may be rooted in the desire to reduce employee medical insurance premiums, whereas another company may provide a wellness program for its employees in an attempt to reduce employee stress and boost employee morale. These are examples of worthwhile organizational philosophies and desired outcomes. To function most effectively, all administrative planning, policies, and decisions are designed and implemented in direct relationship to the organization's philosophy and goals.

Policy

2. *Administrative activities are rooted in sound organizational policy.* A policy is a formal rule or regulation that governs the operations of an organization. An intramural sports program may have a policy that prohibits current or former varsity basketball players from participating in intramural basketball. A commercial fitness club may have a policy requiring that prospective members obtain written medical clearance before being allowed to enroll in a high-intensity exercise class. An athletic training program may have a policy that prohibits athletes from receiving whirlpool treatments without staff supervision. Each of these is an excellent example of a sound policy, in that each is designed to ensure the enjoyment or safety of program participants.

When sound organizational policies are in place, administrative activities such as decision-making should be carried out in a manner consistent with existing policy. A student who hasn't played varsity basketball since her freshman year should not be allowed to play intramural basketball. An apparently healthy member should not be allowed to take the high intensity exercise class while he is still trying to get an appointment for a medical exam. A star athlete shouldn't be allowed to be in the whirlpool unsupervised just because "our old trainer let us do it." If a policy is sound and effective, it should be enforced. If a policy becomes ineffective or inconsistent with the philosophy and goals of the organization, it should not be ignored or disregarded. It should be evaluated and revised or eliminated.

3. *Administrative activities reflect a sincere concern for the welfare and dignity of every person in the organization.* It has been said of teachers that "students will never care how much you know until they know how much you care." The same philosophy can be applied to the administrator-colleague relationship. Every administrative policy, plan, and decision affects others in the organization. Administrators who are aware of colleagues' needs and desires and act out of genuine concern for their welfare and dignity will likely have the support and cooperation of their colleagues, even on difficult administrative issues.

4. *Administrative activities encourage the creative input and cooperative effort of organizational colleagues whenever possible.* Teachers, coaches, athletic trainers, fitness instructors, intramural workers, and recreation supervisors will work more diligently on any issue or project in which they have played a meaningful role in its planning. When staff members have some ownership of an idea, project, or program, it not only enhances the effectiveness of the current project but also encourages creative thinking and effort on future issues. Too often, administrators or individual employees lose sight of organizational goals by becoming preoccupied by the nagging question of, "Will I get credit? After all, it was my idea." It is amazing just how much can be accomplished by a group of people when no one cares who gets the credit!

5. *Administrative assignments should be clearly defined and carefully explained.* No sole administrator, regardless of how talented or motivated, can shoulder the entire administrative responsibilities for an organization. Effective administration is a cooperative effort within which tasks are delegated to appropriate staff members or employees.

For example, in preparation for a comprehensive year-end report, the director of a cardiac rehabilitation program may choose to assign specific research tasks to specific staff members. One staff member may be delegated the task of determining the total number of "patient hours" (patient hours = number of patients enrolled throughout the past year × number of hours each participated in program activities). Another staff member may be assigned the task of contacting program dropouts in an effort to determine common reasons for their nonparticipation. Similarly, the director of an intramural sports program may assign one assistant the task of maintaining a running inventory of equipment and supplies, and another assistant may be responsible for maintaining and updating records (eligibility, medical clearance, and so forth) on all students participating in the program.

Regardless of the specific assignments, delegation is necessary and natural to effective administration. Simply delegating assignments, however, does not assure that they will be carried out in a manner that meets the administrator's expectations. To enhance the probability of achieving the desired results from their delegation efforts, administrators must take the time to specifically define and explain the tasks being assigned and the results expected. Too often, employees fail to fulfill delegated responsibilities because they simply do not understand the specific nature of the task or the specific results expected. Whether written or verbal, instructions and expectations must be explicit and are most effective when the administrator presents them directly to the staff member.

Responsibility
Authority
Accountability

6. *Administrative assignments incorporate appropriate responsibility, authority, and accountability.* Few things are more frustrating for an employee than to be delegated a task and the responsibility for its completion without being given the authority to make the decisions necessary to fulfill the assignment. For instance, an assistant coach who is placed in charge of off-season conditioning should be given the authority to establish training schedules, discipline players who violate training policies, and decide what training methods to employ. Without the authority to make these and other critical decisions, his ability to meet the head coach's expectations will be severely limited. Likewise, a physical education faculty member given the responsibility for equipment maintenance, storage, and check-out procedures must have the authority to restrict access to the equipment storage area and to specify under what conditions and by whom equipment may be checked out. Responsibility without appropriate authority is a no-win situation.

Employees who are given the responsibility and authority for carrying out a specific assignment must also be held accountable for their performance. When administrators delegate a task, they should clearly state the level of expectation, and the employees charged with the responsibility for completing the task must understand that they are personally responsible for the quality of their performance. An assistant athletic trainer who is given responsibility for an athletic team (such as volleyball) must be given the authority to provide the necessary athletic training services and must be held personally accountable if the appropriate services are not provided. Strategies for personnel management are discussed in detail in Chapter 9.

OUTCOME-BASED ADMINISTRATION

Administration, whether in business, education, research, or sport, has but one major purpose: to provide effective leadership toward the attainment of organizational or program goals. To this end, all administrative activities should be clearly focused on achievement of the goals or desirable outcomes toward which the organization is moving. In recent years, the term *management by objectives* has been used to describe a conceptual framework within which administrative and management strategies utilize specific performance-based objectives as a systematic means of assessing progress toward the achievement of organizational goals or specific outcomes. Because goals may be easily stated in terms of specific outcomes, a more accurate term for this administrative framework might be *outcome-based administration*. The relationship between performance-based objectives and organizational goals and outcomes is illustrated in Figure 5.1.

Outcome-based administration

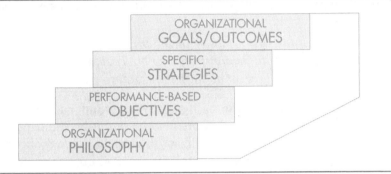

FIGURE 5.1 *Outcome-based Administration Model*

PERFORMANCE-BASED OBJECTIVES

The key to effective outcome-based administration is the design and utilization of specific performance-based objectives. These short-term and long-term objectives may be used as specific markers or indicators by which progress toward organizational outcomes may be assessed.

Writing Performance-Based Objectives

Performance-based objectives (as the name implies) use specific performance indicators to determine the extent to which the objective has been successfully met. Prior to the advent of performance-based objectives, organizational and program objectives were most often stated in rather general and difficult-to-measure terms. For example, a head coach may have had a short-term objective that "my team will be highly motivated and play with few mistakes in the opening game." Or a head athletic trainer might have a long-term objective that "all student athletic trainers will be proficient in basic athletic training skills before graduating from the program." These are both worthwhile objectives. Nevertheless, they are of little practical assessment value because they do not meet the two basic criteria for a good performance-based objective:

Performance-based objectives

1. A good performance-based objective is *observable*.

2. A good performance-based objective is *measurable*.

Although an athlete's motivation, playing mistakes, and athletic training skills can certainly be observed, the above examples are stated so generally as to make observation difficult and measurement impossible.

If written in performance-based terms, these same objectives take on meaningful and usable precision:

> *In the first game of the season, the team will commit fewer than 10 turnovers.*
>
> *By the end of the first semester in the program, each student athletic trainer will be able to demonstrate one NATA-approved technique for taping an ankle to prevent an inversion sprain.*

These objectives are now easily observable and measurable, and, therefore, the extent to which they are met can be easily assessed.

The most difficult aspect of utilizing performance-based objectives is mastering the process of writing performance-based objectives. To be easily observable and measurable, a performance-based objective must contain five specific components:

1. *WHO is to perform the desired behavior or demonstrate the desired knowledge?* The first step in writing a good performance-based objective is to determine precisely who is to exhibit the desired performance. In the above examples, the "who" is represented by "the team" (a collective "who") and "each student athletic trainer" (implying that every student athletic trainer will be expected to demonstrate the skill).

2. *WHAT specific behavior is to be performed or knowledge demonstrated?* Exactly what is to be performed or demonstrated? In the above examples, the "what" is specified as "turnovers" and "taping an ankle to prevent an inversion sprain."

3. *HOW is the specific behavior to be performed or knowledge demonstrated?* This is possibly the most difficult step, as it requires precise language that specifies exactly how the performance will be carried-out. In the above examples, the "how" involves the action verbs "commit" and "demonstrate." In basketball terms, to *commit* a turnover is understood to be any action (other than a rebound) that results in loss of ball possession. When compared with the previous example of a general objective ("to *play* with few mistakes"), it is easy to see the advantages of more precise language ("to *commit* . . . turnovers"). In the athletic training examples, the term "be proficient" is certainly less easily observed and measured than "demonstrate the correct technique" for a precise skill (*taping an ankle*).

4. *Under WHAT conditions is the performance to take place?* This component addresses specific conditions that must be present relative to

performance of the desired behavior or knowledge. Quite often, this refers to a specific criterion condition such as, "On or before June 15, a *written* report must be submitted . . .," dictating that the report must be in *written* form. In the above examples, however, the stated conditions concern precisely *when* the performance is to take place ("*in the opening game*" and "*by the end of the first semester in the program*"). In the athletic training example, "*NATA-approved technique*" also identifies a specific condition by dictating what techniques will be considered acceptable.

   5.   *WHAT CRITERIA will be used to assess the extent to which the objective has been successfully accomplished?* This final component is the key to using performance-based objectives for assessment, because it involves a clear statement of the precise standard of performance that is expected. To quantify statements such as "few mistakes" and "basic athletic training skills" is virtually impossible. By contrast, "fewer than 10 turnovers" and "one *NATA-approved technique*" are easily quantifiable and, thus, easily measurable. If the basketball team in question commits 15 turnovers in the first game, that objective has not been met. On the other hand, if all student athletic trainers can demonstrate one NATA-approved ankle-taping technique by the end of the first semester in the program, that objective has been met.

   The following are examples of performance-based objectives. Can you identify the five critical components in each objective?

1. (Athletics) At the end of the fiscal year, the head coach for every sport will submit a written report reflecting total expenditures within the allotted budgetary resources for that sport.

2. (Physical Education) By the end of the unit on volleyball, each student will be able to serve the ball overhand into the opponents' court with 80% accuracy in game situations.

3. (Athletic Training) Prior to exiting the athletic training room at the close of each work day, each athletic training staff member will enter in the computer all treatment data relative to his/her injury-care work.

4. (Adult Fitness) Each fitness instructor will attend at least one professional update/continuing education meeting, workshop, or conference each year.

5. (Intramural Sports) During the upcoming academic year, 75% of the student organizations on campus will field teams in at least six intramural sports activities.

6. (Recreation) Prior to the first organizational meeting for youth league football, all coaches will have become certified in American Red Cross Basic First Aid and CPR.

Worksheet
Performance-Based Objective

Select a professional area (athletics, physical education, athletic training, adult fitness, intramural sports, or recreation), and write performance-based objectives that contain the five critical components of a good performance-based objective.

Objective #1 _____

_____

_____

_____

Objective #2 _____

_____

_____

_____

Objective #3 _____

_____

_____

_____

Objective #4 _____

_____

_____

_____

Objective #5 _____

_____

_____

_____

Using Performance-Based Objectives

A baseball pitcher who has mastered a variety of pitches must learn how to use those pitches if he is to become successful. In much the same way, an administrator who knows how to develop performance-based objectives must know how to use those objectives to build an outcome-based administrative framework.

1. *Based upon the goals (desired outcomes) of the organization, a comprehensive list of short-term and long-term performance-based objectives will be developed.* Once the goals (desired outcomes) of a program or organization have been identified, short-term and long-term performance-based objectives are written reflecting specific strategies for reaching those goals. Depending upon the size of the program or organization, this "master list" of objectives may be rather lengthy and may require significant time and effort to produce. For this reason, developing objectives may be most effective if this step is approached as a cooperative effort involving all staff members.

Short-term objectives

Long-term objectives

For example, following a meeting in which organizational goals were identified and discussed, the Chair of Physical Education and Exercise Science might delegate to various faculty members the responsibility for writing objectives pertaining to their specific areas of expertise and departmental responsibility. The head of the teacher education (pedagogy) area would write short-term and long-term objectives for the teacher education program, the head of the exercise science education area would write short-term and long-term objectives for the exercise science education, and so on.

2. *Once a master list of objectives has been developed, objectives are grouped into logical and manageable modules or units.* Performance-based objectives should be grouped into logical, functional units to facilitate their utilization. For example, in a physical education and exercise science department, objectives that are relevant to the basic instructional activities program, the professional preparation program in teacher education, the professional preparation program in exercise science, and the department's research program should be grouped under those headings. This enables staff members with primary responsibilities in each of those areas to assume direct administrative responsibility for the objectives that pertain directly to their administrative unit. This is yet another example of encouraging employees to assume ownership of the program or organization based on their specific interests and areas of expertise.

3. *Strategies necessary to achieve the objectives are employed, and the objectives are used to evaluate the extent to which the strategies were successful.* Once short-term and long-term performance-based objectives have been established, specific strategies must be developed for meeting

each objective. For example, an athletics department may be adding a "non-revenue" sport such as men's and women's cross-country. In anticipation of increased budgetary expenditures, the following short-term performance-based objective might be appropriate: *During the upcoming academic year, noninstitutional revenues (funds not provided by the school) will increase by 5%.* As worthy and appropriate as this objective may be, it will be of little value in the absence of strategies for achieving the desired 5% increase in noninstitutional funding. Examples of specific strategies designed to meet the "5% increase" objective are fundraising events such as hosting a county-wide holiday basketball tournament, selling advertising space in football and basketball programs, and a series of weekend car washes conducted by athletes from all sports. The success of the fund-raising strategies may be evaluated quickly and easily by comparing the amount of revenues generated with the criterion set forth in the objective (5% increase).

4. *Objectives and strategies are evaluated on a regular basis, and revised as deemed necessary.* As valuable and important as performance-based objectives and related strategies are to the process of outcome-based administration, they are not carved in stone. Every performance-based objective, along with the strategies employed to meet that objective, should be evaluated carefully on a yearly basis to determine the current relevance to organizational goals and the contribution toward attainment of these organizational goals. Based upon this evaluation, specific objectives and strategies may be retained in their current form, revised to enhance their effectiveness and relevance, or eliminated from the administrative plan.

RESOURCES

Appenzeller, H. T. (1993). *Managing Sports and Risk Management Strategies.* Durham, NC: Carolina Academic Press.

Hall, J. (1988). *Models for Management: The Structure of Competence.* Woodlands, TX: Woodstead Press.

Lewis, G., and H. Appenzeller, (1985). *Successful Sport Management.* Charlottesville, VA: Michie Company.

Railey, J. H. and P. R. Tschauner, (1993). *Managing Physical Education, Fitness, and Sports Programs*, 2d ed. Mountain View, CA: Mayfield Publishing.

Zakrajsek, D. B. (1993). Sport management: Random thoughts from one administrator. *Journal of Sport Management*, January: 1–6.

Zeigler, E. F. (Ed.) (1994). *Physical Education and Kinesiology in North America: Professional and Scholarly Foundations.* Champaign, IL: Stipes Publishing.

The Effective Administrator

6

OBJECTIVES

After studying this chapter, you should be able to:

1. Identify and discuss the characteristics of an effective administrator.
2. Contrast the concepts of strategic leadership and non-strategic leadership.
3. Identify, define, and discuss the three types of critical skills that an effective administrator should have.
4. Identify, discuss, and utilize the "Six Cs" of the conflict-resolution process.

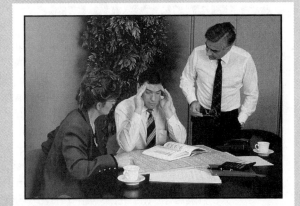

An administrator is typically perceived to be the person in charge of an organization, a program, or some specific segment of an organization or program. Administrators generally have familiar titles such as Director of Athletics, Chair of Physical Education and Exercise Studies, Director of Cardiac Rehabilitation, Head Athletic Trainer, and Director of Intramural Sports. As students view their professional futures, many have difficulty seeing themselves as future administrators, and, therefore, struggle with what they may perceive to be a lack of personal relevance of a professional organization and administration course. Students pursuing a degree in one of the exercise-related professions must understand a key fact about their future role as exercise-related professionals.

*Every member of an exercise-related organization or program **is an** administrator, regardless of his or her specific position.* This is because every teacher, coach, fitness instructor, athletic trainer, and intramural

Administrator

staff member has direct responsibility for some specific segment of the program or organization, even though that segment may be small. Although he or she is not the director, chair, or head, administrative responsibilities are not optional for the exercise-related professional. Therefore, all students preparing to enter the exercise-related professions must strive to develop the characteristics and skills of an effective administrator.

CHARACTERISTICS OF AN EFFECTIVE ADMINISTRATOR

As with great athletes and great statesmen, the well-worn question concerning great administrators is: Are effective administrators born or made? Those who have achieved success in their chosen professions (Michael Jordan and the late Jackie Joyner-Kersey come to mind) appear to perform with such ease that surely they must have been born with exceptional talent — or were they?

Certainly some innate characteristics may contribute to ultimate success in a chosen profession. Physical height is an asset to a person who desires a career in basketball, and an abundance of slow-twitch muscle fibers in the legs will prove beneficial for the aspiring distance runner. Many authorities agree, though, that greatness is determined less by innate gifts than by development of these attributes through rigorous training. The same seems to be true of effective administrators. Success depends more upon the development of desirable administrative qualities than natural gifts and talents. Effective administrators possess most, if not all of the following qualities:

1. *An effective administrator has the ability to think clearly and creatively about complex issues.* Simply stated, one requisite characteristic of an effective administrator is a strong mind. This is not to suggest that all successful administrators are members of *Mensa* (the exclusive society for persons whose measurable intelligence is greater than 98% of the general population — generally IQs of 132 and above). Most administrative work, however, requires significant mental effort (decision-making, planning and organization, and the like), so intellectual strength and creativity are assets important to an administrator.

2. *An effective administrator has a strong academic preparation in one or more of the exercise-related professions.* Administrative leaders in physical education, exercise science, and the other exercise-related professions have themselves been and remain students of their chosen profession. The more knowledge a person has of professional issues, the broader is the perspective that may be brought to bear on administrative issues. In most cases, a program director, chair, and dean holds a terminal

(doctoral) degree in one of the exercise-related disciplines. The head athletic trainer, director of intramural and recreational sports programs, head coach, and director of corporate and commercial fitness programs typically possess a master's degree, and many have terminal degrees. An administrator's professional preparation routinely includes coursework related to issues of organization and administration.

3. *An effective administrator has professional vision.* An administrator without professional vision is like a young child without an imagination. Professional vision is the ability to "see" what is possible 5 years, 10 years, even 50 years into the future. The administrator's professional vision is what shapes the goals and direction of an organization or program. The story is told that upon completion of the Disney World complex in Florida, someone remarked, "Isn't it too bad that Walt Disney didn't live to see this" — to which a relative of Mr. Disney replied, "Oh, he did see it. That's why it is here today." That is the essence of administrative vision.

Professional vision

4. *An effective administrator is willing to exert individual effort to achieve organizational goals.* A common misperception is that administrators plan, supervise, and direct the work of others. Although these duties are important, the difference between ineffective administrators and effective administrators is often the willingness of the latter to roll up their sleeves and work alongside others in the program to reach common goals. When asked what they most respect about their administrator, staff members often state that "he doesn't ask anything of us that he is not willing to do himself" or "she works harder than anyone else in this program."

5. *An effective administrator is a leader.* Programs and organizations look to the administrator to assume the position of leadership, especially on difficult issues. Leadership may be defined as the ability to assume a directing role. As with administrative qualities, leadership qualities can be developed, practiced, and mastered. The particular type of leadership an administrator employs will be dictated, in large part, by the organizational structure within which he or she operates. Some organizations allow, and even encourage, administrators to use *strategic leadership.* Strategic leadership allows the administrator the freedom to make independent decisions and implement personal approaches and ideas. An example is a veteran quarterback who is given permission to call his own plays in a ball game. This example of creative leadership recognizes the quarterback's vast experience and proven expertise in making wise decisions on the field. On the other hand, some organizations require administrators to practice *nonstrategic leadership.* Nonstrategic leadership requires the leader to function according to preestablished guidelines or instructions. The quarterback whose play selection is determined by the coaches on the sidelines is still the leader on the field but is practicing

Leadership

Strategic leadership

Non-strategic leadership

restricted leadership with respect to offensive play selection. Although this practice may have been employed originally to assist young, inexperienced quarterbacks, it is widely practiced today. In much the same way, administrators may be given the freedom to lead creatively, utilizing personal strategies, or may be restricted in the extent to which they may deviate from established guidelines or instructions.

6. *An effective administrator exhibits positive personal characteristics.* Recently, some high-profile professional athletes have engaged in socially unacceptable, even outrageous, behavior, then vehemently dismissed suggestions that they are role models for young admirers. Their denial does not alter the reality that their role model status is not a matter of choice. Likewise, administrators are professional role models, and must accept responsibility for conducting themselves accordingly. Although *professionalism* may be defined in a variety of ways, effective exercise-related administrators offers themselves as a model of professionalism by embodying the following characteristics:

- Honesty, integrity, and loyalty in all personal and professional dealings

- Neat and appropriate dress for specific occasions

- Involvement in professional organizations and activities

- Involvement in community-service activities

- Involvement in continuing professional development activities

- Utilization of grammatically correct and appropriate written and spoken language

- Refraining from the use of tobacco and other harmful drugs

- Refraining from the abuse of alcohol

- Maintaining a healthy lifestyle profile including personal exercise and weight management

Professionalism does not begin when a person enters an exercise-related profession. It begins when the individual becomes a student of exercise-related professions.

7. *An effective administrator possesses and practices strong communication skills.* A popular commercial advertisement suggests that we are judged by the words we use. As stated in Chapter 8, communication is much more than simply exchanging information. The manner in which an administrator, or other exercise-related professional, communicates is a distinct reflection of his or her commitment to professional excellence. Correct spelling, grammar, pronunciation, enunciation, and reading and writing

skills can be learned, practiced, and mastered. Strong communication skills allow administrators to clearly articulate their ideas and concepts and facilitate understanding by people with whom they communicate.

8. *An effective administrator possesses the three major types of critical administrative skills.* Administrative effectiveness depends largely upon the administrator's knowledge, understanding, and application of three critical types of skills.

■ *Professional skills.* Professional skills are specific skills that are directly related to the performance of day-to-day administrative functions. These skills usually are taught as part of the administrator's academic preparation. The following are some typical professional skills: *Professional skills*

budget preparation and management	conflict resolution
	supervision
program planning	program and personnel assessment
scheduling	staffing
facility management	computer literacy
personnel management	

■ *Conceptual skills.* Conceptual skills involve the administrator's ability to visualize and understand the functioning of the entire program or organization, and at the same time to understand the interrelationship of the various components of the program or organization. These skills are not easy to master because they require extensive knowledge of each organizational component as well as a vision of the overall direction of the program or organization. *Conceptual skills*

A good example of conceptual skills in practice may be found in a successful coach. The coach has designed a variety of offensive plays to defeat opponents' defensive efforts. In doing so, the coach has a thorough understanding of how the entire team should execute the play, and at the same time knows precisely each team member's individual responsibility. In much the same way, an administrator should be able to visualize the functioning of the whole program or organization and also know what each staff member and each department must do to attain the organizational goals.

■ *Interpersonal skills.* Interpersonal skills are exemplified by the administrator's ability to work effectively with others toward the attainment of program or organizational goals. A common misperception is that interpersonal skills are limited to getting along with colleagues and relating personally. Although an environment of congeniality is desirable and certainly makes the workplace more enjoyable, collegiality is not synonymous with the concept of interpersonal skills. *Interpersonal skills*

The crux of the issue here is cooperative effort toward attaining common program or organizational goals. As discussed later in this chapter, personal conflicts arise in every organization. The history of sport is filled with examples of teams who fought bitterly among themselves off the field, yet were virtually unbeatable once the umpire yelled, "Play ball!" An effective administrator must have the ability to work effectively with colleagues (including conflict resolution) to maintain progress toward the common goals of the program or organization.

Conflict

9. *An effective administrator is skilled in recognizing and resolving conflict within the organization.* Organizations are composed of individuals with unique personalities, philosophies, and ideas. Therefore, the notion that conflicts can and do arise, even in the most amicable of programs, is not surprising. The ability to recognize and resolve conflicts is among the most challenging of administrative skills.

Conflict recognition

Recognizing what is a conflict requires a basic understanding of the concept of *conflict*. Conflict is not merely disagreement — though disagreement is certainly present when two or more people are embroiled in conflict. *Conflict* may be defined as disagreement that escalates to the point of threatening a relationship. When a disagreement involving personalities, philosophies, or ideas is not resolved easily and quickly, it may continue to grow until the personal or professional relationship of the individuals begins to suffer. When individual relationships suffer, ultimately so does the organization's ability to function productively.

Conflict resolution

Conflict resolution is not something that just happens. It requires conscious effort on the part of all involved parties. Successful conflict resolution is based upon two fundamental concepts: (a) pro-activity, and (b) open, honest communication.

An effective administrator recognizes that, like an open wound, conflict that is allowed to go

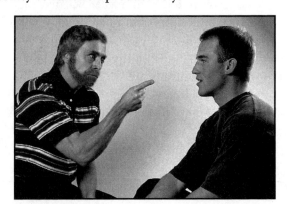

Resolving conflicts inappropriately can lead to stress and anger.

unattended usually worsens. A proactive, rather than a reactive, approach to conflict resolution is essential. Also, both the quantity and quality of communication tend to decrease as conflict progresses. Therefore, open and honest communication is necessary if conflict issues are to be successfully resolved.

THE SIX Cs OF CONFLICT RESOLUTION

The administrator may use the following "Six Cs of Conflict Resolution"as a suggested systematic approach to successful conflict resolution:

Six Cs of conflict resolution

1. *Commitment.* At the heart of every successful program and organization are faculty or staff members who share a common commitment to the goals, and thus the ultimate success, of the program or organization. In many cases, these faculty and staff members also have a commitment to their relationship with their colleagues. When conflict arises, the first step the administrator can take is to encourage those involved to recognize the importance of their common commitment to success of the program or organization and that unresolved conflict is a direct threat to that commitment.

For example, two faculty members in a physical education program may be in conflict over the best strategy for filling an existing faculty vacancy. Although they both agree that the new faculty member has to be capable of directing the program's newly approved sport management program, they are in direct disagreement concerning the qualifications and experience that candidates for the position should have. Faculty member A insists that the position requires an experienced, senior-level faculty member with at least 10 years of experience in directing a sport management program. Faculty member B, on the other hand, believes that a young, junior-level faculty member who has recently received graduate preparation in one of the nation's leading sport management programs would be the best choice. This disagreement has escalated to a point at which the task of writing a position description that will receive full departmental approval seems impossible.

The department chair may decide to meet with the two faculty members to discuss the issue. She may take this opportunity to review the department's earlier unanimous decision to develop a sport management program and reiterate the importance of the new program to continued departmental growth. This is a chance to remind the warring faculty members of the need for shared commitment to what is best for the department. Successful resolution of the existing conflict may depend upon reestablishing a commitment to department goals rather than individual interests.

2. *Communication.* As discussed in Chapter 8, communication is essential in any successful organization. The administrator's task is to facilitate open and honest communication among those involved in the conflict. To continue with the previous example, the meeting of the department chair and the two faculty members should be structured to allow a free exchange of feelings, ideas, and opinions concerning each

faculty member's position on the issue of hiring a new faculty member. The department chair's role becomes that of moderator and facilitator, allowing each faculty member adequate opportunity to identify and explain the ideas and beliefs that define their positions. This is an excellent example of the "all-in-one" principle in practice (see Chapter 8).

3. *Compromise.* Compromise has been described as the failure to hold firm to critical beliefs, selling out or giving in to a position in which one does not believe. This is simply not the case. Compromise is the willingness to set aside one's personal agenda in the interest of the greater good. The greater good is that which is best for the organization. In the example, the department cannot hire a person who meets the specifications set forth by both professor A and professor B. Neither can it hire two new faculty members. Therefore, compromise may be the only viable option. Through the open and honest communication discussed above, an attempt should be made to reach a compromise in the precise candidate qualifications that will be acceptable to both professors.

4. *Consensus.* The goal of compromise is to reach consensus on the strategy for resolving the conflict. As discussed in Chapter 7, consensus is not so much a matter of total agreement of all involved concerning the proposed solution as it is group acceptance that the alternative solution is the best one for the program or organization. During discussion of the issue, the administrator should listen carefully for indications of reaching consensus and be ready to "test for consensus" at the appropriate moment by stating, "It seems that we may be nearing consensus with respect to [a clear statement of the proposed alternative solution]." If all parties respond positively, the details of the compromise can be worked out. If one or more parties indicate that they cannot accept the compromise, however, the administrator may employ one of three strategies.

- The discussion may continue in an attempt to reach consensus.
- The discussion may be suspended, with an agreement to have a future meeting for the purpose of attempting to reach consensus on the issue.
- It may be decided that consensus is not likely to occur, so the administrator must assume responsibility for unilaterally resolving the conflict.

5. *Control.* As mentioned in Step 4, the goal of discussion and compromise is to reach consensus — an acceptable alternative that will bring about resolution of the existing conflict. If consensus cannot be reached, continued discussion may eventually produce consensus. If the administrator senses that consensus is not a viable option, though, he or she must assume personal responsibility by taking control of resolving the conflict through administrative decision.

This step is somewhat of a last resort. Although it will produce a definitive solution, it is unlikely to result in one that has the support of the conflicting parties. Furthermore, one cannot expect an administratively dictated solution to resolve the underlying personal emotional conflict that may exist between the parties. Therefore, every reasonable attempt should be made to resolve the conflict through consensus.

6. *Commitment.* Regardless of the outcome of the conflict resolution process, all parties should exit the process with a renewed commitment to positive collegial relationships and to the goals and ultimate success of the program or organization. In many instances, resolution of organizational conflict is one of the most stimulating, invigorating, and beneficial experiences a program or organization undergoes.

RESOURCES

Appenzeller, H. T. (1993). *Managing Sports and Risk Management Strategies.* Durham, NC: Carolina Academic Press.

Cuskelly, G, and C. J. Auld, (1991). Perceived importance of selected job responsibilities of sport and recreation managers: An Australian perspective. *Journal of Sport Management,* 5: 34–46.

Hatfield, D. B., J. P Wrenn, and M. M. Bretting, (1987). Comparison of job responsibilities of intercollegiate athletic directors and professional sports managers. *Journal of Sport Management,* 1: 129–145.

Katz, R. L. (1974). Skills of an effective administrator. *Harvard Business Review,* 52: 90–102.

Lewis, G., and H. Appenzeller, (1985). *Successful Sport Management.* Charlottesville, VA: Michie Company.

Mullin, B. J. (1980). Sport management: The nature and utility of the concept. *Arena Review,* 4 (3): 1–11.

Tjosvold, D. (1993). *Learning to Manage Conflict.* New York, NY: Lexington Books.

Decision-Making

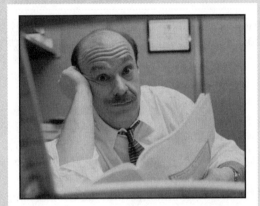

Among the many responsibilities of an administrator, none is more critical than that of decision-making. The ultimate success (or failure) of an administrator is often directly related to his or her ability to make fair, objective, accurate, and effective decisions. Regardless of how simple (the amount of copier paper to be ordered) or complex (the retention or dismissal of an employee) the issue, the final decision, made by the administrator, will have a direct impact on the program or organization.

Decision-making

DECISION-MAKING STRATEGIES

In most organizations decisions are made by a variety of people utilizing a variety of strategies. A head basketball coach may decide which players to start in a given game without consulting anyone else in her program. A head athletic trainer may involve his entire staff in developing the staff work schedule. Most administrative decisions fall into one of three categories, depending upon the specific decision-making strategy employed: autocratic decisions, democratic decisions, and consensus decisions. An effective administrator understands the dynamics of these decision-making strategies and utilizes them appropriately in the decision-making process.

Autocratic Decision-Making

Autocratic decision-making

An autocratic decision is one that an individual makes without input from others. The basketball coach determining her starting line-up without input from others is an example of autocratic decision-making. As is true with all decision-making strategies, the autocratic approach has both strengths and weaknesses.

Autocratic decisions generally require less time than democratic and consensus decisions and reflect the decision-maker's (administrator's) philosophical position on the issue in question. When used excessively and/or inappropriately, however, autocratic decision-making has the potential for undermining the trust necessary for a healthy and productive administrator-staff/faculty relationship. Administrators who make the majority of their decisions autocratically may find that their colleagues begin to feel alienated, unappreciated, and uninvolved. For example, when the program administrator consistently makes important decisions impacting an entire program or organization (curriculum revision, athletic staff meeting times/places, exercise class scheduling, intramural sports activities for the year, and the like) without input from other program participants, it is easy to understand why the staff or faculty may have negative feelings.

Democratic Decision-Making

Democratic decision-making

Contrary to popular belief, democratic decision-making is not simply the process of voting on an issue with the majority opinion dictating the decision. A democratic decision is made by an individual, but only after considering input from other sources. A head athletic trainer would want to consider the class schedules and other time commitments of student trainers before developing a staff work schedule. Nevertheless, the ultimate decision is made by the head athletic trainer.

One of the major advantages of democratic decision-making is that the decision-maker (administrator) has more information (input from others) upon which to base the final decision than is available when making an autocratic decision. This input can be obtained in numerous ways. One of the most common methods of obtaining staff or faculty input on important issues is through open discussion in a staff or faculty meeting. These meetings, with everyone present, affords each staff or faculty member the opportunity to state his or her position on the issue and present information that supports the position. Staff or faculty meetings also provide an excellent forum for *brainstorming* on important topics. Brainstorming is the process of introducing a topic (for example, "How can we offer a wider variety of activity classes with the current faculty and resources?") and encouraging group members to verbalize as many ideas as possible. During the brainstorming session, all suggestions are recorded in writing, with no attempt to evaluate the practicality of each. Once an exhaustive list of ideas has been compiled, the group or the administrator can evaluate, select, and prioritize the most promising ideas.

Voting or *polling* is another popular way to obtain input from colleagues on a specific issue. Whether this is done in a meeting setting or through individual contact, each staff or faculty member is asked to vote his or her preference. The administrator then considers the polling results when making the final decision.

In the process of democratic decision-making, the decision-maker (administrator) is not bound by the results of a vote, although he or she may choose to honor the wishes of the majority when making the final decision. An administrator who consistently makes decisions that are inconsistent with the wishes of his or her colleagues risks losing their trust and confidence and, ultimately, their support.

Consensus Decision-Making

When utilized appropriately, consensus decision-making is a highly effective strategy for making important program and organizational decisions. Of the three major strategies, however, consensus is the most difficult to master, and the most time-consuming, although the results usually are worth the time and effort. A consensus decision is one made by the group (teaching faculty, coaching staff, athletic training staff, aerobics instructors, intramural team captains, and so on), the results of which are acceptable to all group members. On the surface this process may seem cumbersome, time-consuming, and impractical, if not impossible. This need not be the case. Consensus decision-making is successfully used in corporate and educational organizations worldwide, often involving large groups of 100 or more people. To effectively utilize consensus decision-making, several principles have to be understood and practiced.

*Consensus
decision-making*

1. *All group members must be encouraged to participate.* Consensus decision-making is a group process from beginning to end. Therefore, each group member has to understand the importance of his or her contribution to both the discussion of the issue(s) and the decision resulting

from those discussions. The involvement of each group member is more than an opportunity; it is each group member's responsibility.

2. *All group members have equal status in the discussion.* For the consensus strategy to work, the rank, seniority and employment status of group members must be set aside during consensus discussion. This means that the input of a department chair carries no more weight than that of the most junior faculty member, and the opinion of the head coach is no more (or less) significant than that of the newest, least experienced assistant coach. This assures that the group evaluates information and opinions, on their merit, not according to the status of the group member offering them.

3. *The decision-maker's (administrator's) role is that of facilitator.* Unlike traditional decision-making strategies, the administrator's role during consensus discussions is that of a facilitator rather than a director or leader. When directing a staff or faculty meeting, an administrator's position on an issue often receives more visibility and, therefore, may take on added significance from some group members' perspective. When consensus is the goal, in contrast, the administrator must make a conscious effort to facilitate the discussion without assuming a directing role. When he or she participates in the discussion, as explained in Principle 2, the administrator does so as a group member, not as the group's leader. As simple as this may sound, it is often a difficult transition for an administrator to make.

4. *Ideas or suggestions should not be presented for the purpose of playing the role of devil's advocate.* Any group discussion will likely have at least one person who enjoys playing the role of devil's advocate, introducing ideas or suggestions that do not represent his or her honest position but, rather, a position that is likely to produce dissent, and more lively discussion. This is not only time-consuming but often leads the group away from, rather than toward, consensus. Group members' comments should be honest representations of their personal convictions and positions on the issue in question.

5. *The discussion facilitator should know when and how to test for consensus.* When the nature of the discussion indicates that the group may be nearing a common solution or decision, the facilitator may find it helpful to "test" for consensus. To do this, he or she may simply state to the group, "It appears to me that we may be nearing consensus on [a concise statement of the apparent mutually acceptable solution].

For example, an intramural sports director engaged in a consensus discussion with a group of team captains might state, "It seems to me that we may be nearing consensus on scheduling fraternity and sorority games on Mondays and Wednesdays and all other games on Tuesdays and Thursdays." Although this plan may not be everyone's (or anyone's) first choice, the group may have arrived at consensus that it is the best alternative of those presented.

6. *The key to true consensus is total group acceptance, not total group agreement.* For a final decision to be reached by consensus, every member of the group must accept the decision and commit to support the decision. This does not mean that every group member agrees that it is the best possible decision. In the above example, one or more of the team captains may believe that the perfect solution to the scheduling question would be to schedule fraternity and sorority games on Mondays and Thursdays. The discussion, however, may have revealed that such a schedule would eliminate a few teams from the league because of other time conflicts. Therefore, while these team captains may not *agree* that the decision is the best possible one, they do find it an acceptable alternative, and will work to make it successful.

7. *There is no such thing as partial consensus.* What happens when one or more group members cannot accept a potential solution? In the democratic process the decision-maker (administrator) would simply take all the input under consideration, then make a decision. The negative ramifications, however, are clear. Although a majority of the group members may be pleased with the decision and work to support it, those who believe their positions were disregarded are unlikely to enthusiastically support the decision and may even find themselves working in opposition to it. How, then, can this apparent stalemate be resolved? In pure consensus decision-making, a group member who cannot accept a proposed decision has two alternatives. First, if he or she is willing to allow the decision to go forward and can do so without bitterness or trying to sabotage the decision once it is in place, the member may state his or her opposition to the proposed decision but agree to "stand aside." This means that the group member will not block or work in opposition to the decision.

In the second possibility, if the dissenting group member feels so strongly that the decision is wrong that he or she is unwilling to stand aside, this member's responsibility is to "stand in opposition" to the decision. This means that a consensus has not and cannot be reached and the group must either (a) resume the discussion process and attempt to achieve consensus on an alternative decision, or (b) table the issue for discussion and action at a later date. With the latter choice, the dissenting member may be asked to work cooperatively with one or more other proponents of the proposed decision to explore their differences and, it is hoped, reach a mutually acceptable compromise prior to subsequent group discussion and action on the issue. If repeated attempts to reach consensus are unsuccessful, the administrator may have to make a democratic decision in light of the consensus discussions that have taken place.

Although consensus decision-making requires time, effort, and practice, the resulting decisions offer numerous obvious benefits.

- Everyone in the group has played an active role in making the decision, enhancing each member's feeling of self-worth.

- If true mutual acceptance has been achieved, all group members walk away from the process with a certain amount of satisfaction.

- Mutual acceptance of the ultimate decision means that no disgruntled minority has been out voted, and, therefore, is uncommitted to supporting the decision.

A good consensus decision is as near as any program or organization will come to total group cohesion and unity with respect to an important issue.

PRINCIPLES OF DECISION-MAKING

Decision-making begins with knowledge and understanding of the key principles of the decision-making process.

1. *Administrative decisions are based on facts.* The administrator makes a commitment to base all decisions (to the extent possible) on facts rather than opinions, perceptions, innuendoes, or rumors. Although opinions or perceptions may accurately reflect the facts surrounding an issue, they are often tainted with half-truths or even totally false information. Decisions based on half-truths and false information are never good decisions.

2. *Administrative decision-making involves the appropriate decision-making strategy.* Although an administrator may have a distinct leadership style, this does not imply that one decision-making strategy is always better than the others. Effective administrators know that the specific decision-making strategy they select depend upon the specific situation and decision in question. Though autocratic decisions potentially can alienate staff and/or faculty members, some decisions are best handled autocratically. Routine, mundane issues that do not require others' input lend themselves to autocratic decisions. For example, the computerized inventory reveals that the supply of stress-testing electrodes is approaching the reorder level. Does the director of the corporate wellness program have to obtain input from his staff (or have a staff meeting discussion) before ordering a new supply of electrodes?

Also, in rare circumstances an immediate decision is required because time does not allow the administrator to solicit external input. For example, the chair of a physical education department receives a telephone call advising her that a major water main serving her building has broken, flooding the gymnasium. Her autocratic decision to close the facility immediately is probably appropriate.

Most administrative decisions, however, are more appropriately made democratically or by consensus. An example of inappropriate use of the autocratic strategy is an athletic director who changes the men's basketball schedule or makes major budget decisions without input from his staff (coaches, athletic trainers, and so on).

Most successful administrators rely heavily on democratic decision-making. By soliciting input from a variety of knowledgeable sources, the administrator is better prepared to make an informed decision. If financial resources have become available to purchase additional exercise equipment, for example, the director of adult fitness may solicit opinions from her fitness instructors concerning the specific types of equipment they would like to purchase. Based on this information, the administrator can make the final decision.

Some decisions virtually mandate the democratic process. This is especially true of situations in which the administrator has access to information that his staff or faculty do not. For example, several candidates are being considered for a coaching position. Although the athletic staff unanimously prefers a certain candidate, the administrator eliminates the candidate from consideration based upon sensitive reference information that he chooses not to share with the staff.

Consensus decisions are most appropriate when every member of the decision-making group has a similar vested interest in the resulting decision, when each member has valuable information that impacts the decision, and when the group has no clear cut expert on the issue.

3. *Before initiating the decision-making process, the administrator identifies the desired outcome(s) of the decision.* For example, when considering the fate of an ineffective employee, the desired outcome of the administrator's ultimate decision is improved productivity of the program in which the employee works. Therefore, if the employee can be effectively retrained, thereby improving her contribution to the success of the organization, a decision to retain the employee may produce the desired outcome. If repeated efforts to improve the employee's productivity have proven unsuccessful, however, a decision to terminate the employee and hire a replacement may be the most feasible way to obtain the desired outcome.

4. *Regardless of the specific decision-making strategy selected, the administrator utilizes sound problem-solving techniques.* Too often, important administrative decisions are made in a nonsystematic, haphazard manner, and are based on little more than personal experience or opinion. Decisions made in this way are rarely effective and often are damaging to

Problem-solving

the program or organization. For example, the director of an outpatient cardiac rehabilitation program is concerned about steadily decreasing program enrollment/participation and must decide whether to take steps to increase enrollment/participation or to initiate staff downsizing. Certainly past experience and personal opinion will enter into the administrator's reasoning. Even so, thorough understanding and application of sound problem-solving concepts will enhance the probability of arriving at the most effective decision.

STEPS IN DECISION-MAKING

The following constitute the seven basic steps in decision-making.

1. *Identify the real problem.* As simple as this sounds, it is amazing how easy it is to assume that what seems to be the problem is not the *real* problem at all, but merely a symptom or manifestation of the real problem. In the above example, the administrator may assume the problem is simply that fewer and fewer people are choosing to participate in the cardiac rehabilitation program. Actually, the dwindling participation may not be the problem at all. The real problem may be that, following the retirement of the senior cardiologist in the local cardiology practice, the remaining cardiologists are not actively referring patients into the cardiac rehabilitation program. Or the real problem may be that the new YMCA has begun offering adult exercise classes at times more convenient than those at the cardiac rehabilitation center. The list of possibilities goes on.

Until the real problem(s) is identified, any attempt at decision-making will be unlikely to achieve the desired outcome. One of the most effective ways to identify the real problem is to involve staff members in a brainstorming session designed to uncover some likely, though not obvious, *real* problems.

2. *Reject decision-avoidance strategies.* Although not every person is an effective decision-maker, virtually everyone possesses one or more behaviors that may be used to avoid making a difficult decision. People most often learn and practice these "avoidance strategies" early in life. If successful, they continue to use these strategies instead of sound decision-making strategies as adults.

- *Denial* — simply not acknowledging that the problem exists, with the hope that it will vanish.

- *Projection* or *blaming* — refusing to accept responsibility for a problem by shifting that responsibility to someone or something else.

- *Procrastination* — putting off until later decisions that should be addressed immediately.

In many instances, decision-avoidance strategies take the form of alcohol or drug abuse. Regardless of their specific form, all decision-avoidance strategies have several common characteristics. First, they provide temporary relief from the problem. Second, they never solve the problem. Third, their use is potentially destructive to the administrator and the program or organization alike. Effective administrators recognize their favorite decision-avoidance strategies and consciously reject their use in the decision-making process.

Decision-avoidance strategies

3. *Identify potential obstacles to solving the problem.* People rarely make important decisions without encountering opposition. Effective administrators learn to identify potential sources of opposition to various decisions that may result from the problem-solving process. An obstacle associated with many decisions is the need for increased financial support associated with the decision. For example, if it is determined that the steady decrease in participation in the cardiac rehabilitation program is resulting from a shortage of exercise equipment, a decision to add additional bicycle ergometers and treadmills certainly faces the obstacle of additional funding. Obstacles should be identified and addressed before, not after, making a decision.

4. *Identify possible solutions to the problem.* An effective administrator understands that most problems have more than one viable solution, although some solutions will be better than others. Therefore, the fourth step in the decision-making process is to identify all of the available solutions (decisions). Again, brainstorming with selected staff members may be helpful. For example, the primary reason for the decline in enrollment/participation in the cardiac rehabilitation program may be found to be the availability of more convenient and a greater variety of exercise activities at the local YMCA. Before making a decision, the following solutions may be considered:

Revising the program's activity schedule

Hiring additional staff to allow for expanded operating hours and greater variety of activities

Proposing a cooperative venture with the local YMCA

Accepting the diminished role of the program and downsizing the current staff consistent with the reduction in programming

Selecting the *best* solution (decision) is difficult, if not impossible, without first becoming aware of all the viable options.

5. *Evaluate each possible solution.* After identifying all the available solutions (decisions), each has to be carefully evaluated. Some potential solutions are "no brainers" — they simply are not feasible. One possible

solution for the decreasing enrollment/participation problem in the example is to terminate the entire staff, sell all the equipment, and close the program. Although this would surely eliminate any concern about declining participation, it would not achieve the desired outcome of enhanced exercise options for local cardiac rehabilitation patients. Therefore, impractical solutions should be dismissed without further consideration. Solutions (decisions) that are determined to be viable, practical, and potentially effective should be ranked according to their desirability.

6. *Select and implement the best solution.* Several potential solutions may be attractive. Of these, the administrator should select the most promising one and implement it. For example, the administrator believes that the best strategy for increasing enrollment/participation is to offer expanded hours of operation and takes steps to hire an additional staff member and develop a new operating schedule.

7. *Evaluate the effectiveness of the selected solution and adjust it accordingly.* One of the most difficult aspects of administrative decision-making is that no one can know the results and impact of a decision at the time it is made. After making a decision and initiating appropriate actions, the administrator has to monitor and evaluate the effectiveness (results) of the decision. The primary question is: To what extent has the decision produced the desired outcome(s)? If the results of the decision are found to be less effective than anticipated, the administrator must be prepared to make appropriate adjustments. In some cases, fine-tuning the process is sufficient. In the example, this might consist of revising the new operating schedule to provide more evening hours and fewer morning hours. To achieve the desired outcome, however, the administrator might have to select and implement a completely different solution. For example, if expanded program hours fail to increase participation, the possibility of a joint cardiac rehabilitation program with the local YMCA may be considered.

RESOURCES

Browne, M. (1993). *Organizational Decision Making and Information.* Norwood, NJ: Ablex Publishing.

Eden, C., and J. Radford, (Eds.) (1990). *Tackling Strategic Problems: The Role of Group Decision Support.* London: Sage Publishers.

Kleindorfer, P. R., H. C. Kunreuther, and P. J. H. Schoemaker, (1993). *Decision Sciences: An Integrative Approach.* New York: Cambridge University Press.

Nutt, P. (1989). *Making Tough Decisions.* San Francisco: Josey-Bass Publishing.

Rasmussen, J., B. Brehmner, and J. Leplat, (Eds.) (1991). *Distributed Decision Making: Cognitive Models for Cooperative Work.* New York: John Wiley & Sons.

Communication

OBJECTIVES

After studying this chapter, you should be able to:

1. Explain the value of effective communication in the success of a program or organization.

2. Identify and contrast the three types of listening skills that are critical for effective organizational communication.

3. Define the "all-in-one" principle, and discuss its role in effective organizational communication.

4. List and explain the seven specific guidelines for effective organizational communication.

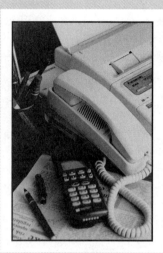

Communication

Communication, according to *Webster's New World Dictionary of American English* (1994), is "a giving or exchanging of information, signals, or messages as by talk, gestures, or writing." As every good administrator knows, though, communication is much more than exchanging information. One might accurately say that effective communication is the stitching that holds the very fabric of an organization together, the foundation upon which successful organizations are built. No single factor is more crucial to healthy personal and professional relationships than open, honest, effective communication.

ORGANIZATIONAL COMMUNICATION

Organizational communication refers to communication among the various parts of a program or organization. The value of effective

Organizational communication

organizational communication cannot be overstated. Just as with personal relationships, professional relationships suffer when the quality or amount of communication diminishes. For example, when teachers or coaches within a department fail to communicate about facility and equipment needs, the result may be needless conflict when two staff members plan to use the same facilities or equipment at the same time. Likewise, a head athletic trainer or intramural sports director who is displeased with the performance of a staff member but fails to clearly communicate these concerns virtually guarantees that the quality of services the program provides will be less than desirable.

To facilitate effective communication and avoid problems associated with poor communication, an administrator should work toward creating and maintaining an environment that values, encourages, and rewards honest, open communication. One of the best ways an administrator can accomplish this is by developing and practicing good personal communication skills. Although all professionals should possess the ability to write and speak clearly and correctly, many administrators, teachers, coaches, sports medicine and fitness professionals, and recreation leaders overlook, and thus fail to develop, good listening skills.

Effective communication is not merely the giving and receiving of information and ideas. It involves understanding, analysis, decision-making, and creative thinking. To that end, administrators must learn the skill of effective listening. Few things will jeopardize internal communication more quickly than the perception that a colleague is not truly listening to the information or ideas a fellow colleague is presenting. Each of us wants the person with whom we are communicating to listen to what we have to offer.

Listening takes many forms. Those most critical to effective administrative/ professional communication are:

Comprehensive listening

Empathetic listening

Critical listening

1. *Comprehensive listening*, comprehending and remembering what is said

2. *Empathetic listening*, listening to and understanding another's concerns

3. *Critical listening*, evaluating content, analyzing points of view, weighing evidence, and making judgments.

A fitness instructor who is having difficulty motivating her students and, therefore, is becoming frustrated with their progress may discuss her concerns with the program director. During their conversation, the administrator (program director) may utilize all three types of listening skills. The program director utilizes comprehensive listening to comprehend and remember the specifics of the instructor's concerns. Empathetic listening allows the administrator to feel the instructor's frustration. Critical listening is necessary for the administrator to evaluate and analyze the instructor's situation and make appropriate, informed decisions and suggestions for alleviating the instructor's frustration. Neglecting any of these listening skills may add to the instructor's frustration. As with any other administrative skill, listening requires commitment and concentration and must be practiced to be mastered.

THE "ALL-IN-ONE" PRINCIPLE

"All-in-one"
principle

Just as poor communication can cause problems, effective communication is a tool for solving problems. Consider for a moment a familiar scenario in which communication is abundant but the lack of *quality* communication is causing a problem. A basketball player complains to the assistant coach that when she runs full-speed, her knee hurts. The assistant coach mentions this to the head athletic trainer, who calls in the player for a conference. Upon examining the knee, the athletic trainer cannot determine the cause of the pain and sends the player to see the team physician. The physician examines the player's knee and discovers a minor problem. He tells her that the injury will respond well to rest and advises her not to practice for the remainder of the week.

After returning to school, the player (who doesn't want to miss practice for fear of losing her starting position) tells the athletic trainer and assistant coach that the doctor told her it was a minor problem that would heal on its own. She does not mention the advised rest. At practice the next day, the player makes several mistakes because of the pain in her knee. The head coach, unaware of the injury, yells at her to "pick up the pace and stop loafing." Finally, the frustrated coach replaces the player on the floor.

After practice, she tells the head coach about the pain in her knee, and the coach immediately sends her to the training room. When she explains to the athletic trainer that the coach sent her, the trainer gives her a note to give the coach, reading, "Amy has had the knee examined by Dr. Harris, and he cleared her to practice and play."

Over the next few days and weeks, the problem becomes apparent, affecting the coaching staff, the injured player, the other team members, and the athletic trainer. The Director of Athletics has received a telephone call from the injured player's parents, advising him of the player's dissatisfaction over her recent lack of playing time. When the Director speaks to the coach, he is informed that she has been injured and the athletic training staff doesn't seem to be effective in caring for the injury. From the perspective of those involved, communication has not been lacking. Figure 8.1, however, illustrates the true nature of the problem.

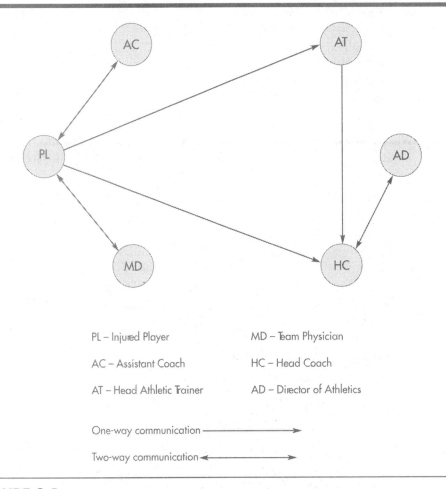

PL – Injured Player   MD – Team Physician

AC – Assistant Coach   HC – Head Coach

AT – Head Athletic Trainer   AD – Director of Athletics

One-way communication ⟶

Two-way communication ⟷

FIGURE 8.1   *Communication Pattern Diagram*

Communication pattern diagram

Using a communication pattern diagram (Figure 8.1) to analyze the communication pattern in this scenario, it becomes evident that the problem is not the result of too little communication but, rather, poor communication among the principal participants. In this situation the administrator should employ the "all-in-one" principle of effective communication: gather *all* the people directly involved in the problem *in one place, at one time*, to discuss *one issue*. In this scenario, the Director of Athletics (as the chief administrator) should schedule a meeting with the head athletic trainer, the head basketball coach, the assistant basketball coach, the team physician, and the player for the sole purpose of discussing the problem. This will give all parties an opportunity to lay all the facts, opinions, and perceptions concerning the issue "on the table" and work cooperatively toward a mutually acceptable solution to the problem. At the very least, open, honest communication can erase misconceptions and misperceptions and, in this scenario, may well pave the way for development of new program policies and procedures for handling such matters in the future.

GUIDELINES FOR EFFECTIVE ORGANIZATIONAL COMMUNICATION

To be most effective, organizational communication must be well-planned, designed to meet the specific needs of the individuals involved, and always in the best interest of the organization. To ensure that these goals are met, the administrator may benefit from establishing and following some specific guidelines by which to carry out organizational communication. The following questions provide the framework:

1. *What type of communication is most appropriate?* In today's world of enhanced technology, organizational communication may take many forms — group meeting, memo, personal conversation, telephone conversation, e-mail, fax, and so on). The specific medium of communication is generally a matter of preference, based upon factors such as convenience, speed of conveyance, number of people involved, and the like. Regardless of the specific medium selected, however, all communication fits into two basic categories or types of communication: formal and informal. *Formal communication* utilizes established organizational lines of communication, focuses on the topic of organizational business, and is initiated and verified in writing, with written documentation retained for future reference.

Formal communication

For example, if the Director of Athletics is concerned about the unusually rapid depletion of departmental office supplies, he may decide that a formal memo to all staff members is the most appropriate way of communicating his concerns. Consistent with the criteria for formal communication, he directs the memo only to those directly under his administrative authority, limits the content of the memo to the office supply issue, and provides, via the memo, a written record of the communication. Formal communication is most appropriately used for all matters of "official organizational business."

Informal communication, on the other hand, often takes place outside of the established organizational lines of communication and typically is based on a less structured relationship of the parties, such as mutual respect, confidence, or friendship. At first thought, informal communication might seem to have little impact on meaningful organizational communication. Informal communication, however, is integral to the total

Informal communication

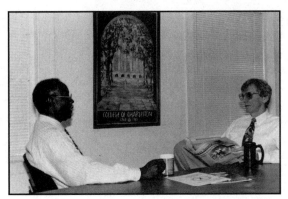

A coffee break presents an ideal time for informal communication.

organizational communication process in that it can allow comfortable discussion of an organizational issue without the constraints of formal communication.

For example, a faculty member at lunch with a colleague may relate her idea for a new course she would like to develop. The feedback gained from this "feeling-out" process may prove invaluable when developing her formal proposal. The value and power of informal communication should not be underestimated.

2.   *What is the main purpose of the communication?* Communication may be used to convey information, request information, initiate discussion and deliberation among colleagues, establish policy, modify a previous communication, and more, but not all at the same time. Too often, a memo or an e-mail message contains so many diverse issues that its purpose is unclear to the recipient. The main purpose of a proposed communication should be clear prior to developing and sharing it.

An athletic trainer who wants to inform all the coaches of a change in training-room hours may choose to have student trainers advise their respective coaches of the new schedule (informal communication) or may believe that a written memo (formal communication) will be more effective. If the decision is to write a memo, it should address the specific issue of the new training room schedule, not present information on a variety of issues, only one of which is the new training room schedule. Stating the purpose of a message clearly and specifically will enhance the likelihood that the message will be read (or heard) and understood.

3. *Is the communication necessary?* Just because an issue is present does not mean that communication has to be initiated. One of the least attractive aspects of administrative work is the immense amount of paperwork and record-keeping. Often the administrator creates needless work for himself or herself and organizational colleagues by calling meetings and writing and distributing memos that are unnecessary. In a relatively small corporate fitness program, a memo to staff members reminding them that the Friday before Easter Sunday is a company holiday and, therefore, the program will be closed is a waste of both paper and the staff members' time. When employees repeatedly receive unnecessary communications, they may fail to properly heed messages that contain important information.

4. *To whom should the communication be directed?* Once it has been decided that communication is necessary, careful consideration should be

given to what specific person(s) should receive the communication. This can be easily determined by asking: Who will be affected by the information? and Who has appropriate reasons for receiving the information?

For example, an Intramural Sports Director deems it necessary to issue a written reprimand to a staff member for consistently showing up late for night games. It may be determined that only the staff member (the person affected) and the Director of Student Activities (senior administrator over student activity programs) should receive copies of the letter containing the reprimand. To make the information available to other staff members would not only be inappropriate but also possibly a breach of confidentiality, which could result in legal action.

On the other hand, the Director of Intramural Sports receives permission to play all intramural tennis matches on the university's varsity courts instead of the city recreation courts as previously announced. This information should be communicated to all staff members, intramural team captains, tennis participants, and anyone else who may be affected by the change.

5. *When is the best time for the communication?* Quite often, the timing of communication is just as important, or even more so, as the nature of the communication itself. When communication involves the announcement or discussion of a significant decision, timing is critical. To call a meeting or issue a memo while information is still being gathered may be premature.

For example, the Director of Cardiac Rehabilitation may be considering a request for expanded hours of operation. While gathering important information (client survey, possibility of hiring part-time staff), he may perceive that the probability of expanding the program's hours is good, and subsequently announce this (either formally or informally) to staff members. After all available information has been collected and analyzed, however, it may become obvious that expanded hours are simply not in the best interest of the program. This apparent change of heart on the part of the Director may result in some staff members feeling misled, and, thus, staff morale may suffer.

On the other hand, if the information-gathering process seems to be taking a longer time than originally anticipated, the Director may wish to provide staff members with one or more status reports on the decision-making process, and an anticipated timetable for its completion. In this way, staff members do not feel left in the dark, and will more willingly accept the fact that the issue will not be resolved as quickly as they had hoped.

6. *What content should be included in the communication?* Ultimately, the true value of any communication lies in what content is conveyed and the worth and appropriateness of that content. Four simple

questions will assist the administrator in assuring that the desired communication is worthwhile and appropriate. *Are other issues related to the central issue of the communication, and, if so, is now the appropriate time to discuss them?* If a Director of Athletics is concerned about the academic performance of the athletes in her program, she may wish to share her concern with the coaches. After gathering information on student athlete gradepoint averages, class attendance rates, and related matters, she prepares a memo to all coaches regarding her concern. Obviously, a number of collateral issues are related to the athletes' academic performance. These include high school academic status of recruited athletes, availability of tutoring and academic skills services, competition schedules that conflict with regular class attendance, and so on. Including a discussion of these (and other) important issues in the current memo, however, may be counterproductive.

If the purpose of the communication is to share her concern along with documenting information, to include the other issues at this time may muddy the water and create a lengthy memo that the coaches may be less likely to read carefully. Instead, a concise memo that gets to the point and includes some hard-hitting specific facts that substantiate her concern may be the most effective way to initiate dialogue, discussion, and eventual resolution.

Does the communication have extraneous content? The effective administrator understands that, with the mountains of paperwork generated in most professional offices, most employees will read first and consider more carefully the communications that the employees perceive as most important. Therefore, as stated above, a concise communication that does not contain unnecessary verbage will be appreciated by those who receive it and will be much more likely to be read.

Could anything in the communication be interpreted as a breach of ethical principles or confidentiality? In announcing to his high school football coaching staff that a fellow assistant coach has resigned and moved to a neighboring community, the head football coach believes his staff has a right to know the circumstances surrounding the sudden resignation. Nevertheless, to provide all the relevant information the coach knows would violate the confidential agreement reached between the school and the former coach.

Does the communication contain anything that may reflect negatively on the institution, the program, or any of the people involved? An old adage states that "a family [organization] should not air its dirty laundry in public." This means that negative publicity concerning an institution, a program, or persons in that institution or program rarely serves a positive purpose. At some point, every athletic program has an athlete who is injured more frequently than others, misses practices because of injury or illness more often than others, and soon develops a reputation as one who uses injury and/or illness as an excuse. Although this is often tempting, an athletic trainer should not communicate her personal negative feelings about the athlete to other staff members, coaches, or players, and certainly not to anyone outside the athletic program. These comments reflect negatively on the program and may even render the institution and program vulnerable to legal action.

Several years ago a well-known professional athlete repeatedly complained of shoulder pain that interfered with his ability to play. Numerous medical examinations uncovered no shoulder injury. As a result, teammates, coaches, and organization officials began to privately and publicly criticize the athlete for his so-called injury. Shortly thereafter, the athlete suffered a career-ending stroke, apparently from an undetected blood clot in the painful shoulder. Communication should not contain any content that reflects negatively on the institution, its programs, or the people in those programs.

Few things reflect more negatively on a program or an administrator than a memo, letter, or posted announcement that contains misspelled words or incorrect grammar. Regardless of their position or title, administrators are professionals, and must communicate in a professional manner. When preparing a written document, an administrator should exercise care to use correct spelling and grammar. If a secretary is to prepare the document for distribution, part of his or her responsibility should be to advise the administrator of spelling and grammatical errors or, with the administrator's approval, make necessary changes. Once the final document has been prepared, the administrator should read and approve it prior to distribution. No administrative written document should be distributed without the administrator's review and approval.

7. *Does the communication include specific expectations, and, if so, are they clearly stated?* A main purpose of communication is frequently to effect some desired outcome. For example, an administrator may ask her secretary or administrative assistant to find out why a piece of ordered equipment has not yet arrived. Although this represents an apparently simple communication, the purpose is clearly to attain a desired outcome (specific information about the delayed delivery). The administrator's expectation may be that the secretary will contact the company immediately, whereas the secretary's expectation is that this matter is not urgent, and can be done later.

As is often the case with miscommunication, the problem is the result of unclear expectations. In this example, the administrator could have prevented the problem by clearly stating her expectations as a part of the request: "Will you please find out why the _____ hasn't been delivered, and let me know what you find out before you leave for the day?".

The quality of internal (organizational) communication is critical to the successful operation of any program. As these guidelines suggest, effective internal communication utilizes the appropriate form (formal or informal), has a clearly defined purpose, is necessary, is directed to the appropriate parties at the appropriate time, contains appropriate content, and includes clearly specified expectations.

RESOURCES

Feldman. E. (1993). Is your department rife with rumors? *Cleaning Management*, February: 62.

Gaskin, L. P. (1993). Establishing, communicating, and enforcing rules and regulations. *Journal of Physical Education, Recreation and Dance*, February: 26–27.

Glenn, E. (1988). Students must listen, communications professor says. *Greensboro News & Record*, February 17.

Golen, S. P., R. Figgins, and L. R. Smeltzer. (1984). *Readings and Cases in Business Communication*. New York: John Wiley & Sons.

Jablin, F. M., L. L. Putnam, K. H. Roberts, and L. W. Porter, (Eds.). (1987). *Handbook of Organizational Communication*. Newbury Park, CA: Sage Publications.

Neufeldt, V. (Ed.) (1994). *Webster's New World Dictionary of American English*, 3d college ed. New York: Macmillan Publishing.

Personnel Management

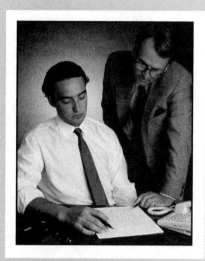

OBJECTIVES

After studying this chapter, you should be able to:

1. Explain the value of the personnel evaluation process to the success of an organization.
2. Demonstrate an understanding of ethical considerations in personnel evaluation.
3. Identify and discuss the three underlying causes of poor employee performance.
4. Demonstrate an understanding of the coaching process and how it may be used to improve employee performance.
5. Identify and explain strategies for removing environmental/circumstantial blocks to effective employee performance.

The most important part of any organization is the people in it. State-of-the-art, high-tech facilities and equipment without qualified, motivated, and committed personnel are useless. On the other hand, highly qualified, motivated, and committed personnel can work together to build and maintain a successful organization, even when facilities and equipment resources are less than desirable. For this reason, each member of the organizational team has to perform his or her responsibilities with professionalism, enthusiasm, and competence. The effective administrator understands the individual responsibilities of each member of the organization, and the interdependent contributions of each member to the success of the organization. When one employee's performance declines, it threatens the success of the entire organization. Therefore, an administrator must establish a systematic plan for personnel evaluation and development if his or her organizational goals are to be attained.

PERSONNEL EVALUATION

Personnel evaluation

No aspect of personnel management causes the administrator more concern than making decisions regarding employee retention, promotions, and salaries. This difficult process can be carried out more equitably and confidently when the administrator follows clearly established, objective guidelines in assessing employee performance — thereby establishing an appropriate database upon which to base decisions. Ideally, employees will perform all their duties in a professional manner, meeting the administrator's expectations. In this ideal world, physical education teachers would always be master teachers, coaches would always have successful programs, athletic trainers would never fail to correctly evaluate and care for an injured athlete, fitness instructors would always individualize instruction to meet the needs of each participant, sport managers would never fail to meet a deadline or attend an important meeting, and recreation leaders and intramural directors would always plan activities with the safety of participants as a primary concern. Exercise-related professions, however, exist in the real world, not in an ideal world, and exercise-related professionals do make mistakes and fail to perform to the expectations of administrators.

Performance appraisal

Ethical Considerations in Performance Appraisal

Any time an employee's performance is assessed, the potential exists for the results to be unfairly influenced by personal feelings, prejudices, and biases. Even the assessment of an employee whose poor performance is virtually certain to result in dismissal has the right, legally and ethically, to a fair and objective assessment. Before performing an employee appraisal, an administrator must make a commitment to conduct the appraisal according to ethical guidelines, outlined as follows.

1. *Know the specific reason for the appraisal.* Employee appraisals are carried out for a variety of reasons. Most commonly they are done to evaluate the employee's performance relative to possible salary increases, promotion within the organization, or to determine whether the employee will be retained or dismissed from his or her current position. The administrator must have a clear understanding of the specific reason that a given appraisal is done and relate this information to the employee whose performance is being appraised.

2. *Make an honest appraisal.* As with quality research, the results of an employee appraisal depend upon the information collected, not on preconceived notions. The administrator must enter the appraisal process with a sincere commitment to perform an honest appraisal, the results of which will be based on objective information.

3. *Base appraisals on information that is sufficient and representative of the employee's productivity*. Appraisal information should be sufficient in scope and depth to provide an accurate picture of the employee's overall performance. Looking at a coach's performance after 1 year provides just a small piece of the "appraisal pie." A coach with a losing record in his or her first season may be unfairly characterized as ineffective, despite positive accomplishments such as expanded school/community interest and improved academic performance of players. Win/loss record is one reasonable criterion for consideration, but a 1-year record is hardly sufficient for assessing the coach's effectiveness. Appraisal data should also be representative of the employee's overall performance. The appraisal of an assistant athletic trainer who has numerous responsibilities should include information on all of the responsibilities, not merely a few. Assessing the athletic trainer's total performance on the basis of his record-keeping skills is not representative of overall performance and is unfair to the administrator and the employee alike.

4. *Make written appraisals available to the employee*. Employees have a right to know the results of all performance appraisals. Providing the employee with an unedited, written copy of the appraisal gives the employee an honest and accurate record of the administrator's perception of his or her effectiveness.

5. *Keep written and oral appraisals consistent*. Divulging appraisal results to an employee is often difficult for an administrator, especially when those results involve unsatisfactory performance. Even so, the verbal comments concerning appraisal have to be consistent with those in the written appraisal. Employees who leave a meeting with an administrator with the perception that their performance is satisfactory may rightfully feel confused if the written appraisal is negative.

6. *Present the results of the employee appraisal as an opinion*. Even at its best, an employee appraisal is based on opinion, because the appraiser must interpret the objective information obtained from the appraisal. An old adage says that "beauty is in the eye of the beholder." This is also true of human performance. Before discussing the details of an employee's appraisal, administrators should point out that the conclusions represent their opinion and professional judgment. To present appraisal conclusions as irrefutable fact allows no opportunity to discuss the employee's perceptions.

7. *Open the appraisal to employee input*. Employees should be afforded the opportunity to provide input into their appraisals. During the meeting with

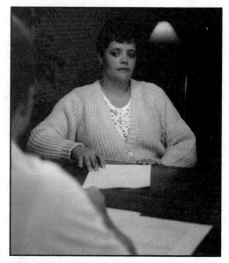

Discussing an appraisal can help the employee make changes that will improve performance.

the appraiser, the employee should be encouraged to ask questions, make comments, and offer explanations or clarification when deemed appropriate. After the appraisal has been thoroughly reviewed, employees should sign the appraisal form, acknowledging the discussion of it and their understanding of (not necessarily agreement with) the administrator's conclusions.

8. *Provide the employee with the opportunity to appeal.* After a thorough discussion of the employee appraisal, the administrator and the employee may legitimately disagree about its conclusions. If that is the case, the employee should be afforded the opportunity to appeal the findings of the performance appraisal in accordance with organizational policy. Prior to ending the appraisal discussion meeting, the administrator should give the employee information about the appeal process and procedural details.

9. *Have a policy concerning the retention and future use of employee appraisals.* Employees who have worked for the same organization for several years may have several appraisals in their personnel file. The organization should have a policy stating how long employee appraisals will be maintained on file (5 years, 7 years, 10 years) and after which a prior negative appraisal will no longer be considered in decisions regarding salary, promotion, retention, or termination.

Determining the Cause of Poor Performance

Before making decisions concerning the poor performance of an employee, the administrator should attempt to determine the underlying cause or causes of the poor performance. Only after the specific cause has been identified can appropriate action be taken to rectify the problem. Just as in the treatment of an illness in which the precise cause must be identified before the proper medicine can be prescribed, the exact cause of poor employee performance must be determined. Without this knowledge, an attempt to solve the problem of poor performance may result in needless retraining of an employee who already has adequate skills or firing an employee for performance problems that are beyond his or her control.

Identifying the precise cause or causes of poor employee performance sometimes is relatively simple. An athlete whose performance fails to meet the coach's expectations, a student whose academic performance is substandard, an employee whose work is unsatisfactory — all share a common characteristic. Poor performance is primarily the result of one of three causative factors:

1. The employee does not know how to perform the task (a *skill/knowledge* or *(S/K)* problem)

2. The employee does not want to perform the task (a *motivation/ incentive* or *M/I* problem)

3. The employee cannot perform the task (an *environmental/circumstantial* or *E/C* problem)

Skill/Knowledge Problem

A skill/knowledge problem is present when a person lacks the expertise, training, or experience to perform the required task(s) satisfactorily. For example, a softball player who repeatedly makes defensive errors may not have received instruction on the proper way to play the defensive position she has been assigned. In the same way, a coach whose team fails to execute fundamental skills may not have the expertise or the experience necessary to teach the skills to the athletes. Employees often fail to meet administrative expectations because of S/K problems. They simply do not have the skills or knowledge, or both to get the job done. The performance evaluation of a fitness instructor who has difficulty maintaining client records may reveal that he doesn't possess the computer skills necessary to operate the new automated data entry/retrieval system.

Skill/knowledge problem

When conducting an employee performance evaluation, the checklist in Figure 9.1 may be helpful in identifying the existence of S/K problems.

If the employee is found to have a skill/knowledge problem, the appropriate solution is retraining. By providing these employees with appropriate training, they will be able to learn the skills and gain the knowledge necessary to successfully perform the desired task(s). For example, an assistant athletic trainer who lacks expertise in proprioceptive neuromuscular facilitation (PNF) techniques might be sent to a PNF clinical workshop to learn and practice the techniques.

Yes	No		
____	____	1.	Is the employee new to or unfamiliar with the task?
____	____	2.	Does evidence suggest a lack of prior training in the task?
____	____	3.	Does the employee have a history of lacking skills or knowledge in previous tasks or jobs?
____	____	4.	Does evidence indicate that the training the employee received did not include an opportunity to practice the skills learned?
____	____	5.	Does evidence suggest that the employee has not received continuing education?
____	____	6.	Does evidence indicate that the employee lacks an understanding of the basic concepts involved in the task?
____	____	7.	Does the task require decision-making for which the employee seems to be unprepared?
____	____	8.	Does the employee have difficulty performing the task correctly even when he/she knows an appraisal is being done?

One or more "Yes" answers indicate that the employee may have a skill/knowledge problem.

FIGURE 9.1 *Checklist: Skill/Knowledge Problem*

Motivation/Incentive Problem

Motivation/ incentive problem

A motivation/incentive problem exists when an employee lacks the interest or desire to perform the desired task(s) satisfactorily. For example, an intramural sports staff member who consistently fails to complete required facility maintenance tasks (taking down nets and standards, returning balls to their proper place in the storage room, and so on) may have the necessary skills and knowledge but may find the task boring and unrewarding. In this example, the employee is performing poorly because of a lack of interest and desire, an M/I problem.

When conducting an employee performance evaluation, the checklist in Figure 9.2 may be used to help identify the existence of M/I problems.

If an employee is determined to have a motivation/incentive problem, retraining this employee will be of little benefit. Improved skills are unlikely to produce renewed interest or desire to perform tasks that employees think are unnecessary or unrewarding. Instead, the appropriate strategy for solving M/I problems is to work with the employee to bring about an "attitude adjustment." These employees should receive counseling and reinforcement that will enable them to change their negative attitude toward the task to a positive one.

For example, a physical education teacher who "rolls out the ball" rather than providing quality instruction may lack the desire to teach, especially if other responsibilities, such as coaching, are more interesting. If the teacher is properly certified, the problem is unlikely to be a lack of skill or knowledge. Therefore, the administrator might meet with the teacher and discuss the specific reasons for the poor performance. If poor pay is at the root of the problem, positive reinforcement may be offered in the form of a salary increase incentive based upon improved performance. Still, though, the administrator might inform the teacher of the observed

Yes	No	
_____	_____	1. Is the task distasteful or perceived negatively?
_____	_____	2. Are others in the organization unaware of the value and importance of having the task done properly?
_____	_____	3. Is there disagreement about the best method for performing the task?
_____	_____	4. Is the effort required to perform the task greater than the rewards received for performing it?
_____	_____	5. Is feedback to the employee lacking concerning the quality of task performance?
_____	_____	6. Does the employee have a history of motivation/incentive problems?

One or more "Yes" answers indicate that the employee may have a motivation/incentive problem.

FIGURE 9.2 *Checklist: Motivation/Incentive Problem*

poor performance, state clear expectations and consequences for not meeting them, and establish a probationary period (as discussed later in this chapter) during which improvement in performance is expected.

Environmental/Circumstantial Problem

An environmental/circumstantial problem is present when employees have the skill/knowledge and motivation/incentive to perform the task but cannot do so because of factors or conditions beyond their control. For example, an exercise science research assistant rarely arrives at work on time. He clearly has the necessary skills and knowledge (knows how to tell time, where to be, and when to be there) and the motivation and incentive (understands the importance of being at work on time and genuinely desires this) to be in the lab at the designated time but is still unable to do so. The problem here may be one of environmental or circumstantial (E/C problem) origin. It may be that another responsibility of this research assistant is to pick up the lab's mail on the way to work and at that time of the morning, lines at the post office are long and slow-moving. Even when the employee is waiting at the post office door when it opens for business, the wait in line results in late arrival at the lab. In this situation the employee's failure to perform satisfactorily is beyond his control.

    When conducting an employee performance evaluation, the checklist in Figure 9.3 may be used to help identify the existence of E/C problems. If the employee is determined to have an environmental/circumstantial problem, neither retraining nor incentives will be productive, because nothing the employee can do will be effective in bringing about a solution. The responsibility for solving E/C problems rests squarely on the administrator's shoulders. In the previous example, the administrator must relieve the research assistant of the responsibility for picking up the mail, change

Environmental/ circumstantial problem

Yes   No

_____ _____ 1. Does the employee answer to more than one superior?

_____ _____ 2. Is the employee expected to "wear many hats?"

_____ _____ 3. Does the position the employee holds have a history of difficulty in meeting deadlines or frequent employee turnover?

_____ _____ 4. Is there evidence of ongoing difficulties with equipment, supplies, unworkable schedules, etc.?

_____ _____ 5. Does the employee clearly have the skills, knowledge, motivation, and incentive to perform the task?

One or more "Yes" answers indicate that the employee may have an environmental/circumstantial problem.

FIGURE 9.3 *Checklist: Environmental/Circumstantial Problem*

the employee's expected arrival time, or accept the conflict presented by the two responsibilities and permit the employee to continue without penalty. When legitimate environmental/circumstantial blocks or barriers exist, the administrator must take steps to remove them.

IMPROVING EMPLOYEE PERFORMANCE

An unfavorable performance appraisal does not necessarily mean that an employee should be terminated. Terminating an ineffective employee and hiring a new employee may seem to be the simplest solution to employee performance problems. In most circumstances, however, both the organization and the employee would be best served by making an effort to improve the current employee's performance, elevating him or her to the desired level of productivity.

First, the process of advertising, interviewing, hiring, and training a key employee is both time-consuming and expensive. A new employee, regardless of how talented and committed, often has to be in a position several weeks or even months before the efforts begin to yield cost-effective results. Second, when the current employee was hired, he or she apparently was considered to be qualified for the position — and more qualified than the other candidates who were not selected. The worthwhile traits that were present when the employee was hired are likely still present and of value to the organization. Therefore, an effective administrator understands and employs sound methods of improving employee performance before giving serious consideration to terminating an employee.

The Coaching Process

Coaching

Although the term *coaching* is usually associated with those who teach, direct, and supervise athletic teams, coaching is really just the process of teaching, guiding, and mentoring someone with less expertise and experience (S/K) or low desire and interest (M/I) for the assigned task(s). Therefore, an administrator engaged in the process of teaching, guiding, and mentoring an employee toward improved performance assumes the role of coach. Although coaching may be effective for resolving S/K and M/I problems, the success of the employee coaching process may be enhanced if the administrator ("coach") will follow a few basic suggestions.

1. *Clarify the employee's assignments.* The organization presumably has employees' assignments listed in a formal position description. In reviewing employees' specific assignments, they can become aware of the precise scope of their performance. This review may reveal a misunderstanding of one or more specific responsibilities by the employee, the administrator, or both. Misunderstandings are common in the absence of

formal position descriptions. For example, an assistant football coach may claim to be unaware that one of his responsibilities includes supervision of student equipment managers. Clarifying this assignment offers an opportunity for the athletic director (administrator/"coach"), head coach, and assistant coach to discuss the assignment.

2. *Clarify specific performance expectations.* The "coach" must explain in detail the quality and quantity of performance expected of each employee. A fitness instructor who regularly cuts classes shorter than the scheduled 60 minutes must be informed specifically that one of the expectations of her performance is that all classes are to be taught for the entire scheduled period except in extraordinary circumstances. Identifying specific expectations will help the employee understand exactly what is expected, and that not meeting those expectations is unacceptable. The administrator should give all employees written descriptions of their specific performance expectations and place a copy in their personnel file.

3. *Identify likely obstacles and roadblocks, as well as ways to get around them.* Few problems are solved without having to overcome a few obstacles along the way. Because of their professional experience, "coaches" may be better prepared than employees to identify some common obstacles before they arise. For example, a physical education teacher may need to attend professional retraining sessions relative to a new, State-adopted fitness curriculum. Because these retraining sessions are held at various locations throughout the state on Saturday mornings, the teacher may encounter problems with travel expenses and having to miss her Saturday morning clean-up supervision responsibilities.

During the initial coaching session, the "coach" should identify potential obstacles and offer possible solutions (such as the opportunity to carpool with other local teachers in order to share travel expenses and reassignment to spring baseball stadium clean-up supervision in place of fall responsibilities).

4. *Clarify your (administrator's) role and contribution to the employee's improvement efforts.* Although the major cause of an employee's poor performance may be related to S/K or M/I problems, E/C problems play a part as well. In the above example, the teacher's lack of expertise and experience (S/K) with the new fitness curriculum requires retraining. Conflicting Saturday morning responsibilities, however, represent an E/C problem. Therefore, the "coach" should support the teacher's efforts, in this example, by arranging a change in the Saturday morning responsibilities. If similar changes are appropriately the administrator's responsibility, they should be identified.

5. *Share relevant personal knowledge and experiences.* Possibly the greatest advantage the "coach" has is professional experience. All administrators have encountered problems and made mistakes during their

professional careers. Employees, however, may see the administrator as the model professional, always making the right move at the right time. The "coach" may find it helpful to relate personal knowledge and experiences relevant to professional performance. All "coaches" have at least one story involving a situation in which they fell short of expectations but, with the help of "coaches," learned from the experience and continued their pursuit of professional excellence.

6. *If needed, arrange for retraining.* When retraining is necessary (S/K problems), the "coach" should take the lead in identifying the types of retraining experiences available and the logistical details (where, when, cost, and so on). The "coach" might discuss with the employee the type of retraining needed and give the employee the assignment of gathering information about appropriate classes, workshops, conferences, and so forth.

7. *Agree to review the employee's progress at suitable time intervals.* The long-range goal of the coaching process is to elevate the employee's performance to an acceptable and productive level. At the same time, short-term goals should be established. The assistant athletic trainer who has neglected her injury record-keeping responsibilities because she is unfamiliar with the new computer system will benefit from having small success indicators or standards on the way to computer mastery. For example, the assistant trainer may be given the following short-term goal: "At the end of the first week of computer training, the assistant trainer must demonstrate competence in entering data (name, date, type of injury, etc.) for 20 players using the new computer system." Frequent assessment of small accomplishments recognizes and reinforces success and enhances the probability of realizing the long-term goal in a timely way.

8. *Establish a probationary period and specify the work to be accomplished during this time.* A probationary period should be established for any situation in which poor employee performance may conceivably result in his or her termination. A probationary period allows the employee time to achieve the desired level of performance, and the administrator a period during which to more closely evaluate the employee's performance. If, following the probationary period, the employee's performance is still unsatisfactory, termination may be the only appropriate option. Prior to initiating the probationary period, the administrator should:

a. Inform the employee honestly and explicitly about the improvement expected so the employee understands precisely what is expected.

b. Allow adequate time for discussion so the employee has the opportunity to explore the total work situation.

c. Encourage the employee to fully discuss any work problems and air grievances.

   d. Plan several short meetings during which interim progress, goal modification, and the like may be accomplished.

   e. Plan for more frequent contacts during the probationary period to facilitate free communication and feedback concerning the employee's work.

Whatever the outcome of the probationary period, the administrator and employee should agree to end the probationary process with mutual respect. At the end of the probationary period, written documentation of the employee's performance should provide adequate information upon which to make an appropriate decision. The report should emphasize and specifically identify the employee's strengths and weaknesses so the employee can use this information in the future.

Removing Environmental/Circumstantial Blocks

As discussed, some employee performance problems arise from circumstances beyond the employee's control. These have to be addressed by the administrator. An intramural sports director cannot conduct a successful basketball program if the school's gymnasium is closed for floor resurfacing. Likewise, an exercise scientist will have difficulty conducting and publishing high-quality cardiovascular fitness research without a good treadmill and supporting data collection instrumentation. Regardless of how well qualified or highly motivated these professionals are, they are unable to perform up to expectations because of environmental/circumstantial blocks (no basketball court and lack of appropriate equipment).

An effective administrator recognizes these environmental/circumstantial blocks and takes steps to eliminate them. The following actions will effectively eliminate many common environmental/circumstantial blocks.

   1. *Provide additional resources.* One of the most common forms of environmental/circumstantial block is inadequate resources. Few exercise-related professionals are fortunate to have positions in which there is always sufficient personnel, money, equipment, and facilities to meet every need. Most teachers, coaches, athletic trainers, fitness specialists, recreation specialists, and intramural directors are skilled at using creative planning to overcome less-than-ideal circumstances. When inadequate resources make expected employee performance impossible, however, the administrator must make arrangements to provide the needed personnel, finances, facilities, and equipment. To the administrator, this may seem easier said than done. The effective administrator, however, recognizes that not to provide the necessary resource support is to deny employees the opportunity to perform their duties as expected.

   2. *Modify employee schedules.* Schedules are developed and maintained so the functions of the organization and its employees can be

accomplished with maximum effectiveness. When schedule conflicts arise, however, the result is often the poor performance of one or more employees, because they simply cannot be in two places at one time. This is also true when personal or family obligations do not conform to the established work schedule.

An assistant director who is in charge of after-school supervision at his recreation center is also a young father. The after-school supervision schedule begins at 3:30, and the employee must pick up his own child at school at 3:30. Therefore, unless some administrative action is taken, the employee will be late. In this situation, the environmental/circumstantial block (the schedule conflict) can be easily removed by modifying the employee's schedule to allow him to begin supervision at 3:45 and scheduling another employee to supervise until 3:45. The employee has no authority to change the work schedule, so the administrator must take action to rectify the problem.

3. *Make needed organizational changes.* Wouldn't it be great if teachers only had to teach, coaches could strictly coach, and athletic trainers could simply care for injuries? The exercise-related professionals rarely have only one responsibility for which they are held accountable. Most wear many hats. The typical physical education teacher may also be a coach, counselor, disciplinarian, club sponsor, clerical worker, custodian, and surrogate parent, and the list goes on. Ultimately, the performance of an employee who has more responsibility than one person can reasonably manage will begin to suffer. Likewise, a coach who reports to two superiors (for example, the director of athletics and the head of the physical education department) may be torn between conflicting expectations of the two administrators.

In both of these situations, the environmental/circumstantial blocks (too many responsibilities and conflicting assignments) can be removed only by administrative action. By revising the organizational plan to relieve the teacher of some responsibilities and place the coach under the direct supervision of one boss, the administrator can enable the employee to become a more productive member of the organization.

RESOURCES

Appenzeller, H. T. (1993). *Managing Sports and Risk Management Strategies.* Durham, NC: Carolina Academic Press.

Friend, J. (1991). *Human Resources in Sport.* Chicago: Nelson-Hall.

Hawkins, J. D. (1996). *The Practical Delivery of Sports Medicine Services: A Conceptual Approach.* Canton, OH: PRC Publishing.

Henry, I. P. (Ed.) (1990). *Management and Planning in the Leisure Industries.* London: Macmillan Education Publishers.

Lewis, G., and H. Appenzeller, (1985). *Successful Sport Management.* Charlottesville, VA: Michie Co.

Management of Fiscal and Physical Resources

OBJECTIVES

After studying this chapter, you should be able to:

1. Discuss the link between sound budget procedures and proper facility planning and management.

2. Identify the three preplanning considerations for budget planning and discuss their impact on the budget planning process.

3. Identify and describe the seven steps of the budget planning process.

4. Describe the difference between short-term and long-term budget plans.

5. Identify five systems of budgeting and compare the advantages and disadvantages of each.

6. Describe the difference between a goal-based system and non-goal-based system of budgeting.

7. Give examples of categories and objects within the line-item system of budgeting.

8. List at least six guidelines to follow when purchasing equipment.

9. List the nine general considerations for facility planning.

10. Select and describe relevant issues in any of the nine general considerations for facility planning.

11. Identify the four major tasks of facility management.

12. List at least three suggested policy guidelines for each of the four tasks of facility management.

T wo closely linked duties of the exercise-related administrator are budget planning and control and facilities planning and management. Even though these two duties have unique characteristics, they combine to form one of the most critical aspects of administration: the management of resources that make possible all programs offered by an organization. (This in no way is meant to diminish the importance of human resources presented in Chapter 9, Personnel Management.) Poor budget planning and control result in inappropriate expenditures and uneven distribution of funds. Poor facility planning and management result in inadequate space, scheduling conflicts, and poorly maintained facilities. None of these is conducive to quality programs.

When budgets are inadequate or poorly managed, facilities are generally the first aspect of the program affected. Maintenance and cleanliness decline and growth is limited, if not absent. And even when the budget is properly managed, it will be strained with unexpected facility maintenance costs or the need for capital outlays to increase space, both indoors and outdoors.

BUDGET MANAGEMENT: PREPLANNING CONSIDERATIONS

Prior to addressing the specifics of planning a budget, some items that affect the way the planner might approach the budgeting process have to be considered: sources of funding, budget periods, and program status.

Sources of Funds

Many organizations must operate from a predetermined budget. For example, the operating budgets of most public schools are determined by the number of students attending the school, or by average daily attendance. (The operating budget is the cost of running the school minus salaries for teachers and staff.) The amount funded for each student is generally determined by the school district after receiving requests from all schools in the district and setting a budget based on expected revenue.

The revenues typically come from a local tax, property taxes in many areas, or lotteries, which now provide the revenue in some areas. The revenue available depends on the willingness of the populace to raise taxes or to buy lottery tickets. The school district establishes its own budget, part of which is the operating budget for the schools. When this money is distributed to the individual schools, the principal has a given amount of money available to allocate to the various programs. Although a small amount of these funds may be shifted between various departments as the school year progresses, the bottom line will not increase.

The physical education program in the school will get some portion of these funds. If the physical education staff has done a good job of selling its program and showing its worth to the overall school program, the administrator may be generous if specific program needs have been justified. If circumstances are not so positive, the allocation may be minimal. Under either circumstance, the amount received is not likely to change. The program must be able to function under this set amount, and planning will be affected accordingly.

The situation is much the same for the intramural program within the public schools, physical education programs, campus recreational programs at public colleges and universities, and municipal recreational programs. Programs funded by governmental grants and corporate fitness and wellness programs that are allocated a lump sum by management operate under the same set of circumstances. Some of these programs have some leeway in raising funds from outside sources to supplement their budgets. They are in essence allowed to generate an income. (See Administering the Budget, below.)

If program income is the basis for the budget, one would think that there would be greater opportunity to manipulate the budget as the program providers desire. This opportunity exists, however, only if the income is available in sufficient quantity. If a program is having difficulty, funds will be short, and this situation will be even worse than working from a predetermined budget.

Even if a program is doing well, income cannot be spent without control. The current year's program budget is generally based on last year's income and, in some cases, on this year's projected income. And what may appear to be a surplus may not be. If the program has grown because of last year's success, expenditures will be higher and the income will be consumed at the same, or maybe even higher, rate. In the case of a surplus, some of this money should be set aside to assure future growth, especially if this growth is likely to result in the need for more costly equipment and facilities rather than constantly plowing it back into programs that might not require increased resources.

Rarely are budgets made for the coming year without giving some attention to current and past budgets and without examining current and past funding sources. Even in organizations that use some form of goal-based budgeting, consideration has to be given to the history of funding and expenditures. This is the obvious place to say, "If we are not aware of the mistakes of the past, we are bound to repeat them." Likewise, if we are not aware of the successes of the past, we are less likely to continue to experience them. Budget planners have to have some idea of the limitations within which they are working. Dreaming about everything you would include in the budget if the money were available is not realistic. A favorite teacher once told me that what physical education needs is more dreamers. He did not say those dreams should be unattainable.

Budgeting Periods

The budget planner also has to be aware of the periods of time for which a budget is made. These can be considered as short-term budgets and long-term budgets.

Short-Term Budgets

Short-term budgets

Short-term budgets are generally considered annual budgets, covering a 12-month period. These budgets provide for the day-to-day operation of a program. Short-term budgets are of two basic types, for which organizations set these limits as a method of control.

Operational budgets

1. *Operational budgets*, including salaries, office supplies, travel and meals, phone, advertising, copying expenses, and the like.

Equipment budgets

2. *Equipment budgets*, covering items that have a predetermined minimum life span, as well as a predefined minimum value. More expensive equipment that is expected to last for an extended period usually requires special budgetary procedures that people at the lower levels of administration do not handle.

Operational and equipment budgets can be, and most often are, handled at the lower administrative levels.

In addition to the typical annual program, an organization may have programs that run for less than 12 months, with funding allocated as needed. Although these programs still have operational and equipment budgets, their period of operation deserves special attention. This is common in athletic and recreational organizations where programs are seasonal. All budgets may be planned and approved at the same time, but funds are released to those running the programs only when the programs are ready to begin operation. This can cause noticeable fluctuations in cash flow within the overall organization and must be taken into consideration during the planning process.

Long-term Budgets

Long-term budgets

Long-term budgets involve budget considerations beyond the annual budget. In organizations that have substantial growth with ambitious building programs, long-term budgeting often cover periods of 5 to 10 years. Although long-term budgeting can involve projections for operational and equipment expenses, they most often deal with *capital outlays*.

Capital outlays

Capital outlays include costs for new indoor and outdoor facilities and renovations to current facilities. They also include expensive equipment that is beyond the limits the organization sets to separate equipment budget items from capital outlays.

Capital outlay equipment is typically purchased through a *competitive bidding process*. This is a requirement for public organizations, and it is also used in the private sector, especially in smaller organizations with smaller budgets that require finding the best deal. In the bidding process, organizations circulate, by mail or advertisement, the description and quantity of the equipment they desire to purchase. Some public agencies have identified specific companies to which they submit bids.

Competitive bidding

When using the bidding process to receive quotes on equipment, detail *specifications* must be included in the bid request. This must be followed up after receiving a response with an offer, to ensure that the offer is being made for equipment that meets the indicated specifications. The bidding process can produce a low price; however, a low price is the *best* price only if the equipment received is the equipment desired. (See Chapter 15, on contracts, for warnings and protections concerning the purchase of goods.)

The bidding process is not limited to capital outlays. Items in the operational budget, such as office supplies and items in the equipment budget, might have low individual costs. When a large number of individual items, such as uniforms for a team or reams of paper for a year's worth of copying, are combined, however, the total is significant and usually will be put out for bid.

Renovation and building projects also utilize the bidding process. Organizations put out bids for architectural firms first. Once an architectural firm has been selected, plans are completed and then the plans are put out for bid. When selecting a building contractor, the same precaution must be taken as when accepting a bid for equipment: ensuring that the bid covers all specifications in the architectural plan. The architect helps ensure this.

Even from this brief description, it should be obvious why capital outlays have to be considered in a timeframe beyond the annual budget. The funds to hire an architect do not magically appear in a budget. The process had to begin some time in the past when needs assessments were conducted and funds were budgeted to initiate the process and carry it through to the stage at which contractors have made bids. Even though the bidding process for contractors was made with some general amount in mind, the budget process now must continue with a set figure on the table. Available funds and funds yet to be obtained must be calculated and worked into budgets — in some cases for years to come.

Many beginning professionals give little thought to capital outlay budgets and expenditures because they see themselves as outside the loop that makes these decisions. This is unfortunate, as their input can be vital to a successful renovation or building program or to the purchase of up-to-date, quality equipment. The new professional often has been exposed to the latest concepts in building design or the newest equipment on the market, either through hands-on experience or through textbooks and current articles. New professionals and all other program providers know what makes a program successful. If they are not being asked for their input, they should be sure to provide it in some way. They can make a significant impact on the use of the organization's resources.

Program Status

The manner in which a budget is developed often depends on its status. Ongoing programs have a history that will influence the planning for the coming year. When the history is positive, planning may be easy and approving funds is not a difficult decision. If the history is negative, however, the program might be facing budget cuts or decreased income, or both, which can complicate budget planning and jeopardize approval of funds at any level.

New programs, on the other hand, have no history. What is planned for them often depends on the success of similar programs within the organization or in other organizations. The planning process for these becomes more detailed. Justification for budget items may now have to be based on research of other programs and may be viewed as speculative by those who are ultimately responsible for allocating the necessary funds. Persons responsible for providing the funds want to know what "proof" is available that this program is worth the expenditure. Especially important here is whether these programs can be offered within the resources currently available. Do they require additional equipment or additional space?

This often gives rise to pilot programs or experimental programs. Even though these programs are considered speculative from the outset, organizations might be willing to appropriate the funds because sufficient evidence is available to indicate that the program is needed and that it will work. Pilot programs might also provide information on the income-producing capability of a program. In addition, these programs are typically of short duration and have less budget expectancy.

Programs that share several of these characteristics are those that have a history but are not ongoing. They are offered as needed or on some type of rotational basis. Examples are recertification programs in fitness organizations, workshops for professionals in the local area, and special topics classes in college physical education programs. These programs are seen as valuable, but they add an expense to the overall budget that has to be justified.

Do enough people need or want these programs to make them worthwhile at a given time?

Have the requirements of these programs changed since the last time they were offered that make them more expensive to offer now?

Do any new requirements for equipment or facilities require significant expense?

Can the current staff still be the program providers or will part of the budget have to go to hire an outside provider?

Questions raised regarding the status of any program will have a significant impact on whether programs are continued or whether new programs are added. The same is true when considering funding sources and budgeting periods. These considerations will be reflected in the budget planning process presented next.

BUDGET PREPARATION, PLANNING, AND PROCESS

As presented by Bucher, budget planning is a continuous process with seven basic steps: planning, coordinating, interpreting, presenting, approving, administering, and appraising.[1]

Planning

This first step involves examining the organizational plan and ensuring that the budget is planned to meet the organization's goals and objectives. The previous discussion related to preplanning. As the planning process begins, these considerations now become part of the thought process of administrators responsible for formulating the budget. Questions of "What has it cost in the past to meet the program objectives?" now become "If we use the past cost as a base, how will it have to change — both additions and deletions — to meet requests for program changes?" Input on these issues should have been provided already by staff members based on their knowledge of program needs. Regular *inventories* of supplies and equipment provide vital information concerning the rate of use of materials, their quality, and the need for replacement.

Surveys of program participants and the community to ascertain interest and needs that the organization can meet should have been completed. They should be conducted throughout the program in the current year to provide input for future budget plans.

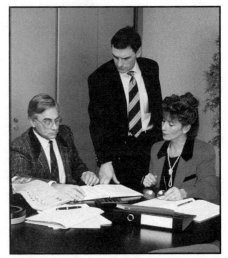

Planning meetings requires research, coordination and a team effort.

If this is not accomplished, the program becomes stagnant, and by the time funds are requested, the program is dead.

This planning process also affects and is affected by the *system of budgeting* the organization uses. The type of budgeting system varies with organizations, which choose the system that best meets their needs. At the program level, the budget system is typically dictated by the system the parent organization uses. In some cases, several systems are combined. Following is a brief description of the more popular forms of budgeting systems.

Line-Item Budgeting Systems

Line-item budgeting system

Line-item budgeting is the system most often used. The budget is separated into categories, and each category is separated into objects or line items (see Figure 10.1). The categories and objects are assigned identifying numbers. Each year the numbers are used to assign funds to categories and objects during the planning process and to record credits and debits to the categories and objects as funds are deposited into and withdrawn from the program account. Forms used to order materials identify the category and object by number to ensure that funds are being spent as allocated. What you received in the category this year is what you can expect in the same category next year.

A common line-item category, "Operating Expenses," coincides with the operational budget mentioned earlier. What types of objects, or lines, would you expect to find under this category? If you say office supplies, telephone, copying, and the like, you are correct. If you say salaries — mentioned under the operational budget above — you most likely are incorrect. Most organizations make salaries a separate category with its own line items. Can you think of reasons why this is the common practice?

This budget system is simple and easy to administer and provides for ease of accounting. If the categories are maintained at the organizational level only and not at the program level, however, no one can determine what proportion of any one category each program is using. This makes meaningful analysis of program effectiveness difficult as related to funds expended for each individual program. The cost effectiveness of each program is hard to determine. And one program can easily get a disproportionate amount of the funds.

One way to remedy this is to have individual program providers maintain their own program accounts. Staffs at the lower levels of the organization tend not to like this because they think it should be someone else's job. This attitude is unfortunate, as good budget management, coupled with effective program provision, has a primary influence on future budget allocations.

TABLE 10.1 *Sample Line-Item Budget*

Budget for Fiscal Year 2000

Institution:	Whatsamatter U.		
Division:	Athletics	Division Account:	500
Department:	Sports Medicine	Dept. Account:	510
Director:	S. Pender		

Category and #	Object #	Object Description	Funded
1000 Salaries			
	1001	Staff	$54,000,00
	1002	Clinicians	60,000.00
	1003	Graduate Asst.	15,000.00
	1004	Work Study	5,000.00
2000 Operational Expenses			
	2001	Office Supplies	5,000.00
	2002	Telephone (base)	1,500.00
	2003	Telephone (long distance)	600.00
	2004	Copying	2,400.00
3000 Equipment			
4000 Maintenance			
		Total Budget:	_____

Incremental Budgeting Systems

Incremental budgeting has as its base the line-item system. The main difference in this system and the line-item system is that the planning process assumes a specific increase or decrease in overall funds available to the organization. Based on this specified amount, each category is increased or decreased proportionately. If the organization is an income-producing organization and expects a 10% increase in income for the coming year (with no increase in new programs), existing programs would receive a budget increase of 10% for each category.

Categories are given as the area in which the increase is generally recognized. This allows administrators some leeway in shifting funds at the object level. If a 10% increase is not needed in phone expenses, for instance, the increase could be used elsewhere within the category. This

Incremental budgeting system

ability to designate funds to various objects during the budget planning process might be even more important when the incremental change is in the negative direction. Some items are capable of being reduced to minimal amounts, thereby allowing the program to survive by maintaining funding levels for the more critical components of a program.

The advantages and disadvantages of this system are similar to those of the line-item system. An additional disadvantage is that each gets the same incremental increase regardless of the program's effectiveness. This could be disconcerting to staff members whose programs are accounting for the increase in funds that makes the positive increments possible. Of course, those who are holding their own during the bad times may feel the same way when they have to experience an incremental decrease because certain programs are causing the organization to lose money.

Formula Funding

Formula funding

Mention was made above of public schools being funded based on average daily attendance. This is an example of formula funding. In this system of budgeting, a formula is used to relate funding to some characteristic of the organization being funded. The characteristics usually are related to production of programs within the organization. This system is typically used when a central body or agent is responsible for distributing a finite sum of money to a variety of organizations — such as schools within a school district. Many states also use this system to fund public colleges and universities.

A disadvantage of this system is that no two institutions are alike and, therefore, no single formula can ensure that each institution gets the funds necessary to adequately fund its programs. Attempts are made to correct this shortcoming by adjusting the formula for the various types of institutions. When formulas are used for colleges and universities, different weightings are placed in the formula for a college that is primarily a teaching college than those that are used for a research-oriented university. For such a system to work, budgets must be based on statistics from the preceding year.

For example, a State's fiscal year might run from July 1 of one year to June 30 of the next year. The State must approve its budget prior to July 1. This requires institutions to turn in their budgets by early spring. To accomplish this, budgets must be formulated in the fall based on the preceding year's statistics. Therefore, budgets approved for 1999–2000 are based on statistics from 1997–1998. Note that no advantage is given for this system.

Planning-Programming Budgeting System (PPBS)

Planning-programming budgeting system

The PPBS system is *goal-based* and focuses on planning and programming. It is most appropriate for large organizations such as governments and the military. This system was first used in these organizations when the public started to demand an accounting for the expenditure of public funds. The purpose of this system is to justify every expenditure. It is advantageous because it takes the focus off individual expenditures; however, it is also a drawback because the process takes a significant amount of time and can be expensive to implement.

In a simpler form, this system can be used in exercise-related programs. Rather than going through the typical step-by-step process of developing a rationale for every program and every expenditure within that program, the budget planner can relate expenditures to specific objectives in the program. If program developers have used a goal-based model such as the behavioral objective model for planning, it is not difficult to relate requested expenditures to the goals and objectives formulated during the planning process.

Zero-Base Budgeting

In the goal-based system of zero-base budgeting, each year's budget is considered to start at zero with each requested expenditure justified by the goals for the coming year. Do you remember the disadvantages of the line-item and incremental systems given above? The zero-base system was instituted to help overcome these problems. Every program will not get X amount just because that is what it received last year. Every program will not get a 10% increase just because a 10% percent increase in income is expected next year. With the zero-base system, every program starts at the same point, zero, and must justify its requests for the coming year.

Zero-Base budgeting system

In this system each program (or division, or department) presents its program plan and states how it will contribute to the overall objectives of the organization. A cost-analysis is given, showing how expenditures are related to the accomplishment of the program and, therefore, to the organization's objectives. Individual programs are then prioritized and budget decisions are made as to the level of funding for each program. If the system works correctly, poor or declining programs will be phased out or dropped and programs that are producing will grow and improve. This is the primary advantage of the system.

The reality is that it is difficult to ignore the past. Planners tend to base their requests on what the program has received and what they expect to receive. This system is goal-oriented and, therefore, much like the PPBS. This makes it time-consuming and expensive and reduces the chances that small organizations will use it.

Coordinating

The second step in the budget process is simple in theory but may not be so simple to accomplish. The theory is that administrators are to integrate and coordinate suggestions from staff, participants, and the community in a way that will match available funds to budget requests to meet the organization's goals. The administrator is dependent on receiving suggestions and recommendations, and depends on these being reasonable and the requests being realistic and justifiable. If they are not, coordination becomes difficult. Administrators are left to make decisions on their own as to what program best meets what objectives.

Interpreting

In the third step the administrators are responsible for communicating budgetary plans to the various programs/divisions. Additional input is requested at this stage, before final decisions are made. Building a consensus for the budget is important at this point. If disagreements arise as to how the budget is to be allocated, now is the time to make them known. Simply saying, "I don't like it" is not enough. Alternative suggestions for the allocations must accompany the disagreement.

Presenting

In presenting the final plan, every attempt should be made to make the presentation as clear and concise as possible. There should be no hidden expenditures. Graphs, diagrams, and the like should be used to simplify and not to confuse.

Approving

Approval of the budget is a management decision alone. There is no vote by the staff. If people at the lower levels of administration have done their tasks properly, everyone should have had an opportunity for input supporting their individual programs. If administrators at the top levels have performed their tasks appropriately, everyone should have had the opportunity to see how their program requests fit into the big picture and, it is hoped, have some understanding of why the budget was formed as it was.

Administering

In the sixth step the administration implements the budget and ensures that appropriate accounting procedures are followed as funds are distributed to each program or charged to program accounts. In situations where programs are allocated a set sum that provides for all needs of the program, this is a relatively simple task. As the program providers need supplies and equipment, they typically complete a *purchase requisition* and submit it to a purchasing office, which procures the goods. When outside services are needed, the program providers follow a similar procedure. When capital outlays are included in the budget, the bidding process and negotiations are handled at the upper levels of administration. Rarely do the program providers handle any funds. In addition to requesting funds, their main task is to review periodic budget reports and verify the accuracy of the charges made to their accounts.

When programs are income-producing and rely on the income to run the program, the procedure becomes more complicated and the program providers are likely to be more involved. Budget control now becomes a process of crediting income to a program's account and debiting expenditures. Program providers are typically responsible for collecting money, providing receipts where appropriate, and transferring the income to the organization's accounting office or business office. Funds are then assigned to the program's account to cover its expenses.

In some cases, programs are given a base account and then are required to raise additional income to support their program. This is typical in public high school athletics, in which the school district provides sufficient funds for basic operation of the program but the athletic department is expected to supplement the budget for anything beyond the basics. Traditional sources of income are *gate receipts, concessions, fund-raising events,* and *activity fees.* Charges for admission to games and activity fees will increase as the program needs increase or as allocated funds decrease, or both.

A relatively new method of raising funds for high school athletic programs is the *pay-to-play policy.* Students wishing to play on an athletic team must pay a fee. This is not unlike income-producing policies of public recreation programs. Some believe that, because these are school activities and school is free, the activities should also be free. This policy has been challenged in court and the courts have upheld this policy as an income-producing policy provided (1) the fee charged is reasonable, (2) disadvantaged youths (those who are financially unable to pay) are exempt, and (3) fees are used solely to cover program operation costs on an equal and fair basis.

Of course, high school athletic programs are not the only programs that have to raise additional funds to meet their needs and improve their programs. Physical education and recreation/intramural programs at the public-school level and in colleges and universities must do the same. Municipal recreation programs must supplement their programs as well. Typical ways of raising funds include fundraising events, fees for memberships, and seeking contributions and grants.

In many situations, income that a program produces is not used specifically to fund that program. In these cases the income is placed in the general budget of the organization rather than into a program-specific account. Money in this account then is made available as needed to the various programs within the organization.

In addition to handling income during this administrative step, it is important to establish reliable procedures for purchasing the material needed for the programs. Railey[2] suggests the following as purchasing guidelines:

- Base purchasing on program needs after conducting an inventory.

- For large purchases, use competitive bidding to get the most for the available funds.

- When purchasing, make product safety an overriding consideration.

- When purchasing agents are not available, delegate purchasing responsibility to competent and interested staff.

- When purchasing equipment and supplies, consider service and replacement of the items purchased.

- Purchase items well in advance of need.

- Ensure that product specifications are written specifically.

- Purchase products at the lowest cost available without sacrificing either safety or quality.

- Do not accept gifts and favors from sellers.

- Ensure that the needs of the disabled are considered when purchasing.

- Purchase only from reputable vendors.

- Purchase from local vendors when possible.

Appraising

Even though it is listed last, appraising is not a final step. Rather, it is an ongoing process performed throughout administration of the budget. Everyone on staff should take an interest in ensuring that the budget is functioning as it was intended. This is accomplished every day through *informal methods* such as *daily observation* and *personal checklists* kept by program providers. The accounting office employs more formal methods in the form of *cost accounting records and reports*, *audits*, and s*taff studies*. Appraisal of the budget serves the same purpose as evaluation for programs. It indicates what is working and what is not. It shows where changes are needed, and it provides valuable information for the next budget-planning period.

Today, programs of any type are expected to be cost-efficient. Program providers are expected to present programs of high quality, and they are expected to use their funds wisely. This can be accomplished only through proper budget planning and sound fiscal management.

FACILITY PLANNING AND MANAGEMENT

As mentioned, facility planning and management can consume a large portion of an organization's budget. The expense is well worth it because poorly constructed and poorly maintained facilities result in an environment that is not conducive to enjoyable participation. People simply will not attend programs in facilities that they think are unsafe, unattractive, and unclean. In situations where the participants have no choice but to attend, as in school physical education programs, the participant's desire to participate and learn can be affected negatively by an environment that is unsafe, unattractive, and unclean.

When facilities are first being planned, adequate funds must be appropriated to ensure safe, quality construction that is attractive and easy to maintain. Once the facilities are constructed and in use, adequate funds must be appropriated for their cleaning and maintenance. Even though quality construction is expected to last, any facility, especially those in the exercise-related professions, deteriorate over time. The higher the use, the quicker the deterioration. Walls have to be repainted, floors have to be resurfaced, racquet court walls have to be resurfaced, fields have to be resodded, pools have to be drained and repaired, showers and locker rooms have to be sanitized, and the list goes on.

Students in the exercise-related professions often question why they must study facility planning or draw a facility plan as an assignment in an organization and administration course. They think the likelihood that they will ever be involved in the actual planning and construction of a facility is remote. Chances are, though, that they will be involved in planning a facility. Even if they are not, knowledge of facility planning will help them understand why the facilities in which they will work are constructed as they are. More important, it gives them insight into making the best use of the facilities as they exist and will encourage them to maintain the facility for optimal use.

Basic guidelines for facility planning and management are set forth next. In reality, these tasks are much more detailed than presented here. Entire books and lengthy manuals have been prepared on the subject. Several of these sources are given in the resources at the end of the chapter. The information presented here serves as a starting point.

GENERAL CONSIDERATIONS FOR PLANNING EXERCISE-RELATED FACILITIES

Facilities should be capable of meeting the goals of the organization and the needs of program participants. Facilities must be constructed with the goals of the organization and its subunits in mind. For example if a university is building a physical education facility to house its physical education and exercise science majors' program, it cannot just build a gymnasium. The gymnasium must be an instructional gym, not just a gym for participation. It must have adequate classroom space and laboratories for exercise physiology, motor development, and biomechanics. It must have isolated areas for individual screening and testing when privacy is necessary. It must have dance studios, weight rooms, swimming pools, racquet courts, running tracks, faculty offices, and the list goes on. The fact that this institution has a program for future professionals in physical education and exercise science indicates that it has goals aimed at developing professionals who can function in the exercise-related professions of tomorrow. Otherwise, the program would not have been approved. The goals of such a program cannot be met in a gymnasium built for playing basketball only.

The same is true for any exercise-related facility. A fitness center that claims it is helping the community move toward accomplishing the goals of *Healthy People 2000* cannot do so with nothing more than a weight room or aerobics studio. If the fitness center has more modest goals but has small facilities in which even the smallest groups feel cramped, it cannot meet its goals. Corporate wellness programs cannot meet their goals of employee fitness if all they have is a classroom to provide lectures. Athletic trainers cannot meet the goals of a growing athletic program if their training room consists of a large storage closet with one wrapping table and an ice machine.

Quality construction and safety considerations should be "job one" in facility planning and construction, while ensuring cost-effectiveness. No one should cut corners in construction. Sufficient funds must be acquired to build the best facility possible. If organizational goals are too ambitious and require a facility that is more expensive than can be afforded, the goals should be reviewed and altered. Then the best facility possible should be constructed to meet the new goals. Cutting corners to get everything you want is likely to result in a substandard facility.

Meeting local codes for electrical standards, fire safety, emergency access, and access for people with disabilities is expensive. Meeting construction standards for heating and cooling systems, lighting, toilet and drainage systems, acoustics, and traffic flow is expensive. Special facilities such as indoor running tracks, swimming pools, and racquet courts are expensive.

Racquet courts provide a good example of the problems created by cutting corners. The wall surface of courts for racquetball, handball, and squash must stand up to a great deal of pressure. Balls and racquets are constantly striking them. People with large, sweaty bodies are continually running into and kicking them. The composition and coatings for these walls are expensive. If cheaper, lower quality materials are used, the maintenance and repair will be constant and the cost of maintenance and repair eventually will exceed the initial cost and continued maintenance of a quality wall. Quality facilities that are safe and inviting, although not cheap, generally result in some reduced cost in the future.

Costs can be contained in certain areas. Combining areas that require major water supply and drainage is a typical cost-cutting measure. To place the men's showers and toilets at one end of the building and the women's showers and toilets at the other end is not economical. Likewise, soundproofing walls is expensive, and often ineffective. Separating noise-producing areas from areas that require quiet is likely to result in reduced cost.

A recent practice of some school physical education and municipal recreation outdoor facilities, in an effort to cut cost, is not to fence these areas. This is a mistake. It significantly increases the likelihood of injury at these sites. Fences help to control the flow of traffic into, out of, and around these areas. When fences are not installed, it is too easy for non-participants to enter the playing area. It is too easy for participants on adjacent fields to run into one another. Time is wasted in controlling who should be on the field and who should not, and with keeping track of those who should be there but are not. The potential negative results of this practice far outweigh the money saved by this corner-cutting maneuver.

Facilities should be planned for multipurpose use. Organizations can no longer afford to build single-use facilities. Gymnasiums must be built for more than just basketball. They must be used for volleyball and badminton as well. They must be capable of being converted into areas for convocations, assemblies, exhibits, and so forth.

Time-sharing by various groups must be considered. Facilities shared by a school and a recreation department eliminate duplication and save taxpayers money. Doubling the use of a facility, of course, puts more emphasis on the need for quality and safe construction. It also requires these two entities to work together in developing their goals and in developing cooperative agreements for use, maintenance, and payment of expenses.

Facilities should be placed in areas that do not interfere with other activities of the organization. Of particular importance to schools, activity areas such as the gymnasium and playing fields produce a great deal of noise and should not be located near classrooms, offices, or libraries. The same can be true in any facility that combines activity areas and meeting or classroom space. If these facilities cannot be placed in separate buildings, every effort should be made to situate the areas as far apart as possible in the same building. In multi-story facilities, classrooms and offices never should be placed under gymnasiums, dance studios, weight rooms, and the like. If an architect says that soundproofing will block the noise, it doesn't.

Facilities should be easily accessible. When you are trying to encourage people to join programs and become more active, you do not want them to be stymied when they are trying to find their way to a certain area. This is one of the most overlooked aspects of facility planning. People who think that they have to negotiate a maze every time they want to use the weight room or swimming pool will quickly lose interest in participating. When access to one area requires crossing another area, activities are constantly interrupted. Participants in the activity that is interrupted are upset, and the person causing the interruption is upset. Both will lose interest.

Accessibility also applies to the positioning of separate facilities. This is of particular importance in school settings where the outdoor areas must be easily accessible from the indoor physical education area. Outdoor facilities should be as close to the gymnasium as possible to prevent loss of time in moving from dressing rooms and classrooms to the field and to facilitate supervision by the teacher during this movement. Barriers such as trailers used as classrooms, maintenance sheds, drainage ditches, and parking lots should not block access to these areas.

Parking lots are a particular problem, as they pose a safety hazard where pedestrian traffic flow would be forced to cross vehicular traffic flow. This is a problem in any organization that has parking adjacent to its facilities. Physical education programs, municipal recreation facilities, corporate fitness facilities, athletic facilities at all levels, and fitness centers — all must be aware of the traffic flow patterns they create. Unfortunately, problems are created in an attempt to make the facilities more accessible to vehicular traffic. This might be understandable when someone has to be delivered to a facility for rehabilitation; otherwise, priority should be given to pedestrian traffic flow. Parking and traffic flow should be kept away from buildings and fields, even if this means a little longer walk after parking the vehicle. After all, we are addressing access to "exercise-related" facilities.

Ease of access also pertains to *access by emergency personnel.* Exercise-related facilities are areas where accidents and injuries are likely to occur. Emergency personnel have to be able to reach all of these areas, both indoor and outdoor, with ease. Signs that are easily noticeable and indicate routes to the various areas of a facility increase accessibility.

Facilities also must be *accessible to people with disabilities*. Even though most exercise-related programs are subject to federal and state laws requiring access for people with disabilities, all organizations should include this consideration in their goals. It is no less important for people with disabilities to be active than it is for the populace at large. Ease of entry at doors and gateways encourages them to enter exercise-related facilities. If this first barrier is not removed, accessibility of the interior of the facility makes little difference. Once in the facility, there should be no barriers to any area. Doors should be wide enough to accommodate wheelchairs and should open easily — or automatically, if possible. Elevators should be present in multi-level facilities. Special equipment, such as lifts, should be available to allow placement and removal of the individuals with disabilities into swimming pools. Wheelchair viewing areas should be available at athletic venues. And, of course, restrooms and showers have to accommodate those with disabilities.

Facilities should be planned so they can be easily supervised. When indoor and outdoor facilities are some distance apart, those responsible for supervising movement from one area to another are at a disadvantage. This is especially true with a group of children being moved. The problem is exacerbated when there are places to hide along the route. Again, indoor and outdoor facilities should be kept close together, and should be open.

Another aspect is the ease of maintaining a secure environment, both indoors and outdoors. Open, well-lit areas enable supervisors and security personnel to have unobstructed views of the area. If facilities are to be used at night, lighting is especially important. The exterior of buildings should have as few indentations as possible, as these areas create dark spots that even the best lighting might not overcome.

Plans should ensure ease of cleaning and maintenance. Ease of cleaning and maintenance depend a great deal on the types of materials used in the building and the interior design of the building. Field layout and construction also contribute to maintenance. Floors should be easy to clean while meeting the specifications for their area. For example, swimming pool decks must be a nonslip surface such as concrete or porous tile. These areas prevent slipping but require special attention to keep clean. Basketball courts can be hardwood or rubberized, but both present special cleaning needs. If hardwood courts are not cleaned daily, sand and grit will wear them down faster. Special water-based cleaners also must be used to prevent slippage. Rubberized surfaces are typically less of a problem, but they mark easily and require special equipment to remove the marks and keep the surfaces clean and attractive.

Gymnastics rooms, weight rooms, aerobic dance studios, indoor running tracks, and wrestling rooms all require special flooring that has its own requirements for cleaning and maintenance. Considering the many different suppliers in the marketplace, choosing the best product is difficult. The best advice is to go with experience, and visit facilities similar to the one you are planning, to see the types of flooring in use and ask questions about its functionality, durability, ease of cleaning, and maintenance.

Floors in non-activity areas may be a little easier to clean and maintain. The key here is that hallways must hold up to heavy traffic flow and regular cleaning. Tile floors with slanted baseboards seem to work best because they tend to be the least expensive, yet attractive. Other surfaces may be more durable but are apt to be more expensive. Carpeting helps to reduce noise but is more difficult to keep clean, especially in areas where spills may occur. Offices and meeting rooms would be the best place for use of carpet. Classrooms present a problem, too. Carpeting helps to reduce noise in these areas but even the best carpet does not hold up well under the traffic in classrooms in educational settings.

The circumstances may be different in noneducational settings. Carpet in therapy settings and athletic training facilities can add to the ambiance of these areas and create a more soothing atmosphere. Client/patient activities in these areas often take place on the floor. Carpeting certainly would be more inviting than most other surfaces. For those who think carpet might add to the growth of germs in these areas, studies have shown that with regular, proper cleaning, this is not the case.

Restrooms, locker rooms, and showers have special cleaning considerations. Showers and locker rooms should be non-slip and well-drained. In the past, these areas were divided from other areas by a lip that prevented water from running into other areas and also allowed the areas to be flooded for easy cleaning. Because these areas should be accessible to people with disabilities, they no longer can have lips. This requires special attention to the construction of these floors to ensure proper drainage and ease of cleaning without causing water problems in other areas.

Drainage also plays a significant role in the care and maintenance of fields used for outside activity. Well-drained fields require less maintenance and can be watered regularly without interfering with use of the fields. Although underground watering systems might add a little to the initial cost of fields, this is money well spent. They save time and provide a better playing surface. Artificial surfaces once were very popular for outdoor areas, but more injuries and high maintenance and replacement costs have caused these surfaces to lose favor. Artificial surfaces, however, are still popular for outdoor tracks.

In addition to the floors, the walls of indoor facilities should be given consideration in relation to ease of cleaning. Walls should be smooth, with few or no ledges. Walls and coatings on those walls should stand up to repeated cleaning, especially in areas where large groups gather. Inevitably the walls will be leaned against, bumped into, and marred by items that people carry in crowded areas. In areas where equipment is moved about often, the walls should withstand the expected minor bumps without leaving noticeable nicks and gouges.

Wall treatments in some areas can add to the attractiveness of those areas but also can increase the need for cleaning. Mirrors in dance studios, aerobic rooms, and weight rooms add to the room's attractiveness and make it look larger. Also, participants can use mirrors to check whether they are using the correct form when performing exercises. Mirrors, however, have to be cleaned regularly to maintain their attractiveness. If mirrors on one or two walls are sufficient, placing mirrors on all four walls is not necessary.

Facilities should be constructed with expansion in mind. Successful programs typically grow over time. Facilities never should be built simply to meet the number of participants expected during its first year of operation. The facility should be large enough to accommodate growth over the next several years. If facilities are located in growth areas, the initial size of a facility may be difficult to determine. If facilities are built so they can be readily expanded, initial size is not as critical.

"Easily expandable" means that buildings can be added to without much difficulty and at minimal cost. Corridors are constructed such that they can easily lead to additions to the existing building or to new adjacent buildings. Internal and external walls are constructed as non-weight-bearing walls that can be easily removed to increase the size of existing areas. Heating and air conditioning ducts and electrical and water systems are structured so the systems can be easily expanded. In areas where space is limited, buildings are being constructed so they can expand upward by adding floors.

Facility planners must consider the aesthetic appeal of the facility. Architects want their creations to be aesthetically pleasing — to catch the eye and stand out. That is fine, and architects should have some leeway in creating an attractive facility — as long as the creation does not take away from its utility. If funds are restricted, no space can be wasted. This is true for indoor and outdoor areas alike. Clearly attractive facilities attract participants. This is important when the program has to be marketed and income has to be produced. But if the program organizers go deep in debt to create an aesthetic facility that cannot meet the goals of the program, they have made a grave mistake. Aesthetics must always be balanced with utility.

Each of the above descriptions is only a sketch of what actually has to be done in planning a facility. Their purpose here is to give the future exercise-related professional some feeling for the enormity of the task and to have a reference point from which to measure the first facilities in which they are employed.

Guidelines for Facility Management

Students majoring in an exercise-related program of study today are likely to work in any of a wide variety of facilities in the future. These facilities include K–12 physical education facilities, secondary school athletic facilities, college/university physical education and recreational facilities, college/university sports and athletic training facilities, public and private recreation facilities, fitness center facilities, corporate wellness and fitness facilities, wellness and fitness centers in adult living centers, therapeutic facilities in sports medicine clinics and hospitals, and professional sport facilities. There are probably more. These various facilities can be loosely placed into five groups: educational, athletic, recreational, sports medicine, and fitness/wellness.

Facility management

No single set of facility management guidelines would suffice for all of these groups. Even so, some general guidelines would have application for most, if not all, of these facilities. Facility management can be divided into the following tasks: scheduling, supervision and security, maintenance, and custodial care. These activities have to be coordinated to prevent conflict and ensure maximum use of the facility. This is especially important when the facility is used by more than one group within an organization or by totally separate organizations.

People in the upper levels of administration consider themselves fortunate when they have a facilities manager who coordinates all of the management tasks for a facility. In large exercise-related programs, this is a must. In small and even medium-sized programs, it is a rarity. In many situations, a different person from different segments of the organization is responsible for each of these tasks, and the left hand likely does not know what the right hand is doing — and even worse, doesn't care to know. Nothing is more discouraging than to have a program scheduled for a certain facility and to arrive and find that someone else is using the facility, or maintenance is being performed, or cleaning is going on, or the security personnel have taken off early, locked the building, and no one has a key.

Although a policy guide will not solve all management problems, it certainly will help. The main reason is that a good policy guide represents a compromise among all of the people who use a facility and who can affect use of a facility. It is the beginning point for the communication that is necessary to solve conflicts that are common when many groups use the same facility or when different groups are responsible for managing the same facility.

For example, in large organizations in which security is a division within the organization responsible for providing security to all facilities, conflict is unlikely concerning use of the facility. The conflict arises when security does not know anything about scheduling the facility and does not open the facility on time. Security might not schedule extra staff for crowd control at large events. Or security might not schedule anyone on weekends because the facility is not expected to be open. If security is included in making the policy guide, part of the policy is to identify who is to contact security concerning the schedule, who is the contact at security, and how far in advance security should be notified concerning any changes in the regular schedule. In addition, security feels more a part of the facility management process instead of an outsider.

Policy Manual

Following are some general suggestions for a policy manual in each of the four management task areas.

Scheduling

- Identify one person within an organization as the coordinator for scheduling all exercise-related facilities. If more than one organization uses a facility, the persons identified in each organization should serve as a team, but one should still serve as the main coordinator.

- Establish a regular operating schedule for all facilities, indoor and outdoor.

- Establish a procedure for informing all persons affected when schedules must be changed.

- Set priorities for the various groups that use the facilities, indicating changes in priority throughout the day.

- Set schedules for custodial care and regular maintenance functions.

- Establish procedures for dealing with unscheduled maintenance.

- Establish policies and construct forms for lease arrangements and contractual agreements for outside groups and individuals who might use the facilities. (Have these checked and approved by the organization's legal counsel, if available.)

Supervision and Security

- Make a list of all supervisory positions, and delineate the responsibilities of each position.

- Establish a timeframe for walk-through inspections and security checks.

- Establish procedures for recording accomplishment of responsibilities, including notes of walk-throughs and security checks.

- If certain areas of the facility are controlled and can be entered only with a key, establish a policy as to who controls signing in and signing out of keys.

- Establish a policy for who can and who cannot use the facility (include provisions for potential users).

- Establish a policy for entering and leaving the facility, such as a sign-in/sign-out log, and for indicating proof of right to be in the facility.

- Establish policies for monitoring equipment, including check-out and inventory procedures.

- Establish policies for what the facility can and cannot be used for, indicating control factors (do's and don't's) to be in effect when it is used for a given purpose (especially where outside groups are concerned).

- Establish policies for fees for use of facility for all groups (internal and external), if appropriate.

- Establish policies for lease agreements for use by outside groups, if allowed.

- Formulate rules of conduct for all areas of the facility, and post these in conspicuous places within the appropriate areas.

- Establish a procedure for informing all supervisory and security personnel of these rules.

- Establish a procedure for evicting persons from the facility. If reasons other than violation of the rules of conduct or lack of right to be in the facility can result in eviction, ensure that they are designated in the policy.

- Establish a policy indicating when security must be present. (In some facilities, this will be all hours the facility is open for operation.)

- If security is not available at all times, establish a procedure for contacting security when needed.

- Establish a policy that allows for easy identification of supervisory and security personnel, such as uniforms or name tags.

- In large facilities, provide building maps in prominent places near entrances, stairs, and elevators.

- Establish an emergency plan for evacuation, to include posted signs for routes of evacuation.

■ Establish a plan for handling emergency situations in a facility, including the procedures for contacting emergency personnel, for directing emergency personnel to specific locations, and signs that clearly mark the location of various areas of a facility.

■ Include in the policy manual all risk-management procedures established for the facility, and ensure that all personnel have read these procedures.

■ Establish a procedure for recording and filing all accounts of emergencies and nonemergency accidents and for notifying administrative personnel.

■ Establish a policy for scheduling and recording training sessions for all personnel responsible for supervising the facility.

Maintenance

■ Identify equipment and utilities that must be inspected regularly.

■ Establish a procedure for inspecting equipment and utilities including who is responsible for the inspection, and for recording the outcome of inspections and what was found.

■ Establish a procedure for scheduling, completing, and reporting repairs, to include the use of work orders when maintenance is provided by an in-house maintenance section.

■ Establish a procedure for contracting with outside maintenance services when needed.

■ Establish a procedure for handling emergency maintenance situations.

Custodial Care

■ Identify the cleaning and ground-care needs of all facilities, emphasizing areas with special requirements.

■ Establish procedures and methods, including scheduling, for accomplishing all cleaning and grounds-care needs.

■ Establish standards for cleanliness and grounds care, and establish a policy for checks to ensure adequacy of cleaning and grounds keeping.

■ Establish a procedure for notifying custodial services when special cleaning or grounds-keeping services are needed.

■ When outside custodial services are used, establish policies for contractual arrangements, and ensure that all of the above are included.

(Have contracts approved by legal counsel if available; if not available, take necessary actions to retain counsel for such purposes.)

Policy manuals covering management of facilities can be lengthy. Manuals for a given facility may contain fewer or more items than those listed here. Although manuals take time to formulate, they are well worth the effort. Manuals should be reviewed regularly, and altered as management needs change. When a situation arises that is not covered by the policies, the manual should be altered as soon as possible to accommodate the situation.

A well-written policy manual will save time and effort in the future and will help assure that the facility management functions are carried out. When the facility management functions are carried out, use of the facility should be at its best and the use of fiscal resources in relation to physical resources should be most cost-effective.

NOTES

1. C. A. Bucher and M. L. Krotee, *Management of Physical Education and Sport*, 11th edition (Boston: WCB/McGraw-Hill, 1998).

2. Railey, J. H., and P. R. Tschauner, (1993). *Managing Physical Education, Fitness, and Sports Programs*, 2d ed. (Mountain View, CA: Mayfield, 1993).

RESOURCES

Arnheim, D. D., and W. E. Prentice, (1997). *Principles of Athletic Training*, 9th ed. St. Louis: McGraw-Hill.

Bucher, C. A., and M. L. Krotee, (1998). *Management of Physical Education and Sport,* 11th ed. Boston: WCB/McGraw-Hill.

Crompton, J. L. (1995). Economic impact analysis of sports facilities and events: Eleven sources of misapplication. *Journal of Sport Management* 9: 14–35.

Flynn, R. B. (1993). *Planning Facilities for Athletics, Physical Education and Recreation.* Reston, VA: American Alliance for Health, Physical Education, Recreation and Dance.

Leith, L. M. (1990). *Coaches Guide to Sport Administration.* Champaign, IL: Leisure Press.

Mull, R. F. (1997). *Recreational Sport Management*, 3d ed. Champaign, IL: Human Kinetics.

Olson, J. (1997). *Facility and Equipment Management for Sport Directors* (American Sport Education Program). Champaign, IL: Human Kinetics.

Ray, R. (1994). *Management Strategies in Athletic Training.* Champaign, IL: Human Kinetics.

Tharrett, S. J., and J. A. Peterson, (Eds.). (1997). *American College of Sports Medicine's Health/ Fitness Facility Standard and Guidelines*, 2d ed. Champaign, IL: Human Kinetics.

Turner, E. (1987). Facility design, trends and innovations. *Journal of Physical Education, Recreation and Dance* 58 (January): 34–35.

Planning for Program Evaluation

OBJECTIVES

After studying this chapter, you should be able to:

1. Describe the relationship between evaluation and planning.
2. Discuss and explain each step in the evaluation cycle.
3. Develop a goal.
4. Describe the difference between a goal and an objective.
5. List and discuss at least three sources of goals.
6. List the five common characteristics of a goal.
7. Describe the difference between formative and summative evaluation.
8. List and discuss the strengths and limitations of the behavioral objective model of evaluation.
9. Discuss the importance of the validity and reliability of test instruments.
10. Identify situations in which quantitative and qualitative evaluation would be used.
11. Describe the importance of reporting evaluation results.

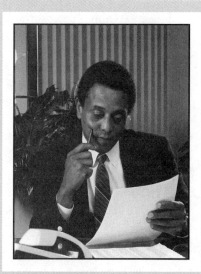

Evaluation is the process of determining progress. It is ongoing. Evaluation grows out of effective planning and, in turn, provides feedback to allow future planning. No other function of management is more critical than evaluation. It serves as a check on all other functions of management. It is used to assess the effectiveness of programs, the performance of staff, and the usefulness of facilities and equipment. It provides support for the things that are successful, and it provides information to support change when change is needed. This chapter addresses program evaluation only.

Evaluation

The process of program evaluation can be seen in a series of questions that are cyclic, ongoing.

1. Are the goals and objectives set during the planning process being accomplished?

2. If the goals and objectives are not being met, why are they not being met?

3. What changes are necessary, and how can they be made?

The evaluation cycle from which these questions arise is depicted in Figure 11.1. Before these questions can be answered, an appropriate planning process must be in place for the selection of goals and objectives.

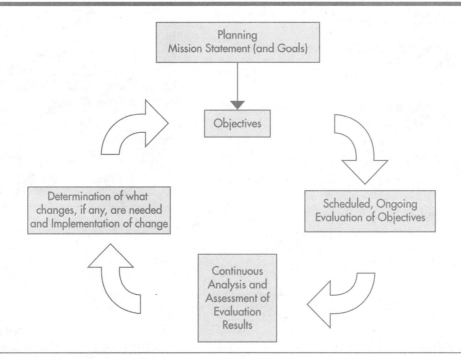

FIGURE 11.1 *Evaluation Model*

SETTING GOALS

Evaluation does not begin when a program is nearing its end and the organization or an administrator decides to perform a few tests to determine what has or has not been accomplished. Evaluation begins when an organization is formed or a new program is added. Evaluation begins with proper program planning. Mission statements, goals, and objectives should be written with evaluation in mind.

Mission statement

When an organization is formed, it is formed with a particular *mission* in mind. An organization's mission is its purpose, its reason for being. A *mission statement* is an expression of this purpose, along with the philosophical view of the organizers as to how they see their organization fitting into the bigger picture and the effect the organization will have on that big picture. This effect should be something that is measurable.

In a small organization, one mission statement usually suffices. In larger organizations with numerous divisions, each division should have its own mission statement. In these cases, the mission statement of a division supports the overall mission of the larger organization.

For example, a large university has a mission that is primarily educational. As part of the philosophical view the mission statement represents, it likely would address the importance of creating and maintaining an environment that is most conducive to learning. If this university considers, as part of this conducive environment, the health and wellness of its students, it is likely to establish a wellness center. The staff of the wellness center then would formulate its mission statement, which would address statements in the university's mission statement. Of course, the wellness center could add other points to its statement as long as these statements do not conflict with the mission of the institution.

Mission statements serve as the primary *goal* of an organization. Goals are general statements concerning desired outcomes in a program. They may be short-term or long-term. No specific time period delineates a difference between short-term and long-term goals. Short-term goals, however, are more immediate and are expected to be accomplished along the way to accomplishing the long-term goals. Long-term goals are those goals set farther into the future. It is often said that long-term goals are those you will never accomplish but will continuously strive to attain. A mission statement can be viewed as a long-term goal. Success in meeting long-term goals is indicated by success in meeting the short-term goals.

Goals

Short-term goals

Long-term goals

Sources of Goals

Short-term and long-term goals generally come from two sources. They can come from an outside source, or they can come from within the organization. The outside source is typically a professional organization to which professionals in the field look for guidance for things such as meeting current requirements or staying abreast of current trends. In cases in which the professional organization provides *accreditation* to the program or will serve as a *licensing* or *credentialing* agent for those who complete the program, the guidelines of the professional organization become mandatory. There are also cases in which professional organizations recommend that certain guidelines be followed. These recommendations might become mandatory for some programs and voluntary for others.

Public school physical education programs provide an example in which recommendations by a professional organization are becoming requirements. More and more states are adopting criteria established by the National Association for Sport and Physical Education (NASPE) as the standard for what should be accomplished in secondary school physical education programs. Individual programs in states that have adopted the NASPE criteria must include these criteria in their goals. This does not mean that these are the only goals the program has to set, but they must be included. States that have adopted these criteria can now evaluate individual public school physical education programs based on the extent to which they meet the stated criteria. Individual programs can also evaluate themselves based on the same criteria and make changes in their programs if they are not meeting the criteria.

Programs that offer *continuing education units (CEUs)* for various exercise-related professionals must also meet criteria established by professional organizations. These organizations, based on their own goals and objectives, determine what they will and will not accept as program content for renewal of certificates and licenses. They also determine who is qualified to present the content. Organizations that want to sponsor recertification programs would have to have their programs reviewed and approved by the certifying agency. Part of this approval requires them to have goals that are compatible with the certifying organization. Once the programs are in place, they would become part of the evaluation process of the organization presenting the recertification program. Attracting participants to the program, success of the participants in the program, and program evaluations and recommendations by the participants would all play a part in evaluation.

Some programs must set goals that address needs specified by law. Educational programs that receive federal funds must comply with Title IX of the Educational Amendments Act to the Civil Rights Act of 1964. Exercise-related programs that are non-private and in which persons with disabilities are likely to participate must comply with the Americans with Disabilities Act of 1990. Chapter 14 provides further discussion on laws that affect planning in various organizations.

Some organizations do not follow any specific guidelines from professional organizations. These organizations determine their own goals. Even in these situations, the organizations might be influenced by guidelines from professional organizations, but they have no obligation to make them part of their program goals.

For example, no one tells private fitness centers that they must set a goal of enrolling a certain number of members. This goal is driven by economics and the desires of the owners as to the size of the center they believe they can support. The owners initially determine what can be done. In the future, the owners might work with the directors and staff to modify current goals and set new goals.

An example that should not be overlooked is one that falls somewhere between goals resulting from guidelines from professional organizations and self-determined goals. On some occasions guidelines result from national initiatives in various areas. Exercise-related programs are fortunate to have several initiatives in their area. Excellent sources of goals for a wide-variety of exercise-related programs are *Healthy People 2000: National Health Promotion and Disease Prevention Objectives* (1991) and *The Surgeon General's Report on Physical Activity and Health* (1996). The U. S. Department of Health and Human Services does not mandate that any specific program meet the goals expressed in these two initiatives. Individual programs are free to use them or ignore them.

Whether goals are taken from an outside source or developed in-house, they must be realistic, reasonable, challenging, achievable, and quantifiable.[1] The first four of these characteristics depend on the nature of the organization formulating the goals. What is realistic and reasonable for a program offered on a grand scale where money is no object will not be realistic or reasonable for a small program with limited funds. On the other hand, small programs may have little or no trouble finding goals that are challenging, whereas the larger programs might have difficulty finding new goals that continue to elevate the program to a level the staff considers challenging. Regardless of the size of the program, the goals must be achievable, or at least continuous progress toward the goals must be achievable.

Each of these goal characteristics is linked to evaluation. "Achievable" would seem to be the one most closely linked. If goals are realistic and reasonable, though, they should be achievable — unless, of course, the staff hired to conduct the program is incapable of doing so. In either case, achievable goals, like realistic, reasonable, and challenging goals, are tied to the nature of the organization. The fifth characteristic, quantifiable, is the one most closely tied to evaluation. Whether a goal is or is not quantifiable has nothing to do with the nature of the organization. A goal is quantifiable if it is measurable or if it at least

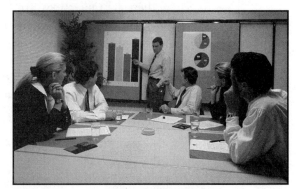

Visual aids can assist in establishing goals.

can be broken down into parts that are quantifiable and, therefore, measurable.

Mico's model for health education planning indicates that measurability is part of the first step in a five-step process for goal setting.[2] The five steps are:

- Establish criteria for goals. As an example of criteria, goals must be measurable events, and they must be framed in a reasonable time.

- Ensure that goal setting is linked to the organizational or community policy development. This is important because policy is the driving force behind the organization of systems necessary to carry out the plan.

- Make a comprehensive statement of alternative goals and the effects or consequences of each. This requires the ability to project into the future to anticipate changes that are likely to occur.

- From the list of alternatives, select goals to pursue. Several models of decision making can be applied to this step. Mico strongly recommended total group support in decision making. (See Chapter 7, on the decision-making process.)

- Develop strategies for implementing goals.

The method used to establish goals should predetermine the strategies for implementing them. The quantifiable aspect of goals, if met as a criterion, should reveal a series of steps that, when accomplished, should lead to meeting the goal. These steps are called *objectives*. Figure 5.1, in Chapter 5, depicts the link between goals and objectives.

Linking Objectives to Goals

Goals express the purpose of an organization and how that purpose will be accomplished through its programs as delivered to a given audience or audiences. Objectives are the steps to be followed to meet these goals. They must be stated in observable terms that can be easily interpreted and followed by the persons responsible for presenting the programs.

Objectives
Provider
objectives
Performance-
based objectives

Objectives can be stated in terms of the persons who deliver the program (*provider objectives*), or they can be stated in terms of the audience and what is expected of the audience during and after program presentation (*performance-based* or *behavioral objectives*). Provider objectives serve as guides detailing a stepwise procedure to be followed by the program provider. These objectives can be in the form of checksheets — of particular value to persons new to a program. Evaluation of this type of objectives can provide valuable information for determining whether the procedures were or were not followed correctly when attempting to reach a goal.

Provider objectives should be written only after the performance-based objectives have been written. Performance-based objectives are the key to successful evaluation. Whereas provider objectives establish a checklist which, if followed, can guide the provider in doing exactly what he or she needs to do, performance-based objectives provide a checklist for program evaluation. A well-formed performance-based objective includes *the content to be presented* and *the behavior expected of the participant* once the content has been presented. The content is derived from the goals, which have been established previously.

The behavior is the change that is expected to take place in the participant as a result of experiencing the program. The change expected might be determined by the persons formulating the goals and objectives, or it might come from outside sources. The change might be related to:

1. Obtaining knowledge (cognitive)
2. Performing physically (psychomotor), or
3. Changing attitude or feeling (affective).

Performance-based objectives should be written in a precise form that indicates the type of change expected. Procedures for writing performance objectives are presented in Chapter 5.

DETERMINING METHODS AND PROCEDURES FOR PROGRAM EVALUATION

As presented in Chapter 5, management by objectives, or outcome-based administration, is standard procedure in many organizations. For this to take place, reliable information must be provided through evaluation. Once the performance-based objectives are written, appropriate methods of evaluation must be selected, procedures must be administered effectively, and an analysis must be done. This process should begin early in the planning stages and involve everyone who will be effected by the evaluation.

Types of Evaluation

Evaluation is typically of two types: formative and summative. These are defined as follows:

1. *Formative evaluation*: Provides immediate feedback during program planning and implementation to improve and refine the program. Evaluation information is collected from a variety of sources both before and during program implementation.

Formative evaluation

2. *Summative evaluation*: Determines achievements, such as numbers of individuals who changed their behavior or whether other program objectives were reached. It is conducted at the end of the program.

Other terminology, including *process evaluation* and *outcome evaluation* have more recently appeared in the literature. Even though they have slightly different definitions, they are not noticeably different from formative and summative evaluation.

Evaluation is an ongoing process. Formative and summative evaluation combine to do this. Those who seek methods of evaluation for their programs will choose formative evaluation to determine preprogram status and ongoing evaluation during presentation of the program, and they will choose summative evaluation to determine the overall results of their program. That is the easy decision. The more difficult decision is choosing the types of evaluation instruments best suited for collecting formative and summative data.

Evaluation Models

The methods chosen for collecting data depend on the model of evaluation that has been chosen during the planning process. The model advocated in this chapter is the performance-based *behavior objective model*. This model requires the establishment of predetermined goals and objectives. Meeting these goals and objectives determines the productivity and overall success of the program. In essence, performance-based objectives become the *standard* for measuring success of the program.

Success can be indicated by change in the participants in the program or accomplishment of those administering the program. Change in participants would be indicated by things such as an increase in knowledge about fitness for students in a physical fitness unit or improvement in range of motion in an injured elbow joint following rehabilitation. Accomplishments of those administering the program could be indicated by increasing enrollment in a fitness center by 50% or by having an athletic budget in which expenditures do not exceed income at year's end.

The behavior objective model has the following strengths and limitations.[4]

Strengths:

- It is objective. The values of the evaluator do not interfere with the outcome of the evaluation.

- The goal is predetermined. The evaluation is based on whether the goal was or was not met, not on whether it was appropriate.

- The goal can be expressed as measurable objectives. This makes it easier to determine whether the goal was or was not met.

Limitations:

- Because the goal and objectives are preset, they might represent the values and interests of persons (such as the funding agency) rather than those directly involved in the program.

- Only those items included in the objectives are evaluated; therefore, other positive outcomes of a program will not be identified or evaluated.

There are other evaluation models. The behavior objective model was chosen as the only model to be presented here because of its role in the cyclic process of planning and the direction it gives for evaluation to those involved in presenting the program. The limitations listed above for this model can be overcome by ensuring that everyone involved in the program is involved in creating the goals and objectives and by assuring that the objectives cover all aspects of the program. This can be time-consuming, but will be well worth the effort when it results in goals and objectives to which everyone in the program believes they have made a personal contribution.

Evaluation Methods

Performance-based objectives indicate the demonstration of a certain behavior or the presence of certain conditions before a program, during a program, and after a program has been conducted. Because of this, evaluation instruments must be valid and consistent in assessing pre- and post-program conditions, sensitive enough to indicate incremental changes during the program, and tailored to the content of the objective.

Validity is an important concept in evaluation. Valid instruments measure what they were intended to measure. Validity is broken down into the following forms.   *Validity*

1. *Content validity.* The instrument measures all of the content areas in a program. If a test that covers only certain areas of the content presented in a course is used to measure change in knowledge, the test does not have content validity and, therefore, does not adequately measure the effect of the program. If a questionnaire does not collect information on all characteristics of an individual that might affect his or her performance in a program, it is not a valid instrument.

2. *Criterion-based validity.* The instrument accurately depicts the relationship between two measures. If the relationship is to be established between two criteria in the present, an instrument that accurately does this has *concurrent validity.* If an instrument accurately relates a current

criterion to a future criterion, it has *predictive validity*. In the first case, current knowledge about cardiovascular disease risks is related to current smoking practices. In the second case, weakness in muscles surrounding the knee joint might be used to predict certain types of knee injuries in soccer players. In both of these cases, the instruments used must have both criterion-based validity and content validity.

3. *Construct validity*. The instrument accurately measures psychological constructs such as locus of control of reinforcement or self-efficacy. These instruments are of value in behavioral-change programs in settings such as fitness/wellness centers, where program providers are interested in predicting success in the program based on scores on these instruments. These instruments have to be constructed by experts in these areas and tested for validity.

Reliability

Reliability refers to the ability of evaluation instruments to provide consistent results each time they are administered. Reliability depends on each of the following:

1. *Stability reliability*. The evaluation instrument consistently gives the same results, or nearly the same results, each time it is used. The theory here is that if an instrument is used today to measure a certain characteristic in an individual or a group, and then is used 2 weeks (or any reasonable time) later to do the same thing, the results should be the same provided nothing has happened to affect the characteristic being measured. If an instrument meets this standard, it is assumed be reliable across groups as well as within groups. This procedure is considered a test-retest method of establishing reliability.

2. *Internal consistency*. Each item of the instrument measures some part of the total picture that is being evaluated, and results on each item are correlated to results on the evaluation as a whole. If the total results of a pre-knowledge test are in a medium range but one group of questions has a high score and another group of questions has a low score, the test instrument does not have internal consistency. Instead of measuring knowledge that has some relation to the questions, the test is apparently measuring knowledge in two separate areas.

3. *Inter-rater reliability*. Evaluation instruments should yield the same results regardless of who administers the instrument. Evaluation results also should be the same within groups and across groups. This is particularly important when data are being collected by observation or by use of a rating scale. Ease of understanding the instrument and ease in administering the instrument are aspects of inter-rater reliability. For example, if two teachers are using the same rubric to assess the skill level of the same players while participating in a five-on-five basketball game, their ratings of the two players should be the same or nearly the same.

Validity and reliability of instruments are always important in evaluation, and they become even more important when the results of evaluation are reported to outside sources. If, for example, one of the reasons for evaluation is to provide data to an outside source that will use the data to determine whether to continue to fund the program, the evaluators will emphasize the validity and reliability of their evaluation procedures. They may be required to include statistical procedures used that support validity and reliability statements.

When using evaluation results for in-house purposes only, formal statistical methods are less likely to be used. In those cases, persons who are responsible for evaluation could easily put less emphasis on validity and reliability of the instruments they use. This would be a mistake. If evaluation is to have meaning, it must be used to effect change. If the instruments used are not valid or reliable, something may be changed when it is not necessary, and, more important, change may not be made when it is needed for program continuation and growth.

Methods of Data Collection

The selection of evaluation methods is a crucial part of the planning process. The administrative considerations in this process include:

- cost of evaluation instruments
- ease of administration and the resulting time involved
- overall usefulness of individual evaluation instruments
- number of people needed to administer certain instruments
- appropriateness of the method for large or small groups or individuals
- preferences of methods of those responsible for evaluation
- availability of standardized and pre-made methods
- ease of interpreting and reporting the data collected.

These considerations often have to be weighed against one another to select the best method of evaluation.

In some cases, this aspect of planning may be relatively straightforward. For example, teachers may be expected to use standardized tests to ensure that certain criteria are being met. The costs of the tests are predetermined. Who administers the tests, when the tests are administered, and how the results are reported may also be predetermined. Planning becomes a matter of budgeting for and ordering the tests and scheduling the test administration, collection, and reporting.

In other cases, the planning has to be done from the ground up. There may be an overall general plan for evaluation with each program provider responsible for developing the specifics for his or her individual program.

The program providers are free to select or develop their own evaluation methods as long as these methods accurately assess the changes the programs are expected to bring about.

Deciding as early as possible in the planning process whether evaluation will be primarily quantitative or qualitative, or both, is important. The *quantitative* approach is deductive in nature and produces data such as counts, ratings, and scores. Evaluation that is quantitative is generally considered *objective*. The score on a knowledge test following an instructional unit or the increase in number of repetitions in an exercise following rehabilitation are quantitative results. Quantitative evaluation is used in programs seeking specific changes such as increased number of participants, decreases in number of days absent from work, changes in heart rate resulting from exercise, changes in pre- and posttest skill tests, and so on.

Quantitative evaluation

The *qualitative* approach is inductive and is used most often in evaluations involving descriptions, opinions, and attitudes. The following are some uses of qualitative evaluation:[5]

Qualitative evaluation

- describing individual outcomes
- understanding the dynamics and process of programs
- obtaining in-depth information on certain clients or sites
- focusing on the diversity of clients or program sites.

Because qualitative evaluation deals with opinions and attitudes, it is considered *subjective*.

Many programs involve both quantitative and qualitative elements and, therefore, require both types of evaluation. A fitness center might be evaluated on a quantitative basis by the number of clients it has. If the numbers are declining, some qualitative data might help to determine why.

Individual evaluation instruments also have both quantitative and qualitative elements. For example, questionnaires can be used to gather specific quantitative information such as demographic data and they also can be used to collect opinions or to assess attitudes. These characteristics increase the usefulness of evaluation instruments.

Evaluation instruments are of unlimited variety. *Standardized tests* are available in many exercise-related areas. This means that the results can be compared to norms for various age groups in each aspect of fitness tested. In the area of fitness testing, for example, AAHPERD's Physical *Best* is widely used, as is the *FitnessGram* provided by Prudential Insurance. Standardized instruments for assessing constructs such as locus of control of reinforcement and self-efficacy are also available from a wide variety of sources.

Knowledge tests, questionnaires, skills tests, checksheets, and the like are discussed and presented in most texts dealing with specific topics and in tests and measurement texts. Specific protocols for evaluating change in injury rehabilitation are available in the areas of athletic training and physical therapy. Specific protocols for assessing cardiovascular functioning pre- and post-exercise training are available for a variety of settings including fitness classes and exercise science lab programs.

When pre-made evaluation instruments are not available or if those that are available do not fit the need of a given program, self-made instruments can be constructed. This is common when questionnaires have to cover material unique to a specific program and when knowledge or skill tests have to cover material in programs created by a certain person. If self-made instruments are to be used where data must be statistically supported, the instruments must meet expected standards for validity and reliability.

Regardless of whether the instruments chosen are pre-made or self-made, they must meet the needs of the program. A standardized instrument should not be selected just because it has been pretested and has a good reputation. If it was developed under conditions different from those in your program, the results will be of little meaning to you. The scope of this text does not extend to the various types of evaluation instruments available and why each is best suited for various situations. That is left for test and measurement/evaluation texts.

EXAMINING AND REPORTING EVALUATION RESULTS

Once the evaluation instruments have been administered and the results collected, they must be examined to determine their exact implications for the program. This examination might be done by the person who administered the instruments, or by someone specifically assigned to examine the results, or possibly by a group of individuals. Regardless of who is responsible for the examination, this person, or these persons, must view the results objectively.

If the examiner is biased and sees in the results only the things he or she wants to see, the evaluation will be of little value to the program. Others will discover the bias. If these "others" are people responsible for providing funding to the program, biased reporting could be devastating. If these "others" are individuals in the program who look to these results to validate their performance and to provide a rationale for change and growth, biased reporting will cause them to lose confidence in the evaluation process. This will affect future evaluations because they will be seen as a waste of time. If evaluation is to foster change and growth, results must be examined for what they are, nothing more, nothing less.

Once the examination of the results is complete, the reports made may be formal or informal. Formal reports typically are made after final evaluation. If final reports must be made to funding sources, boards of directors, stockholders, deans, athletic directors, and the like, the reports are expected to be written and presented in a designated format. These reports are typically quantitative, with emphasis on final figures:

How many passed?

How many failed?

How many attended, and what percentage completed the program?

How many hours were saved as a result of improved work attendance?

These are the types of information expected in such reports. Presenting this information in a clear, concise, and easily readable format is important. In some cases, formal reports are expected to be presented orally. Overheads or slides depicting what is presented in the written report make the presentation easy to follow and can be used to highlight important information.

Informal reports are usually made to the staff responsible for presentation of the program that has been evaluated. These reports are made throughout the program on formative and summative evaluation results. The effective administrator does not underestimate the value of these reports. Those responsible for program delivery often feel left out because communication of evaluation results is only one-way — and that way is not in their direction. Evaluation results must be reported to those who can effect change.[6] Individuals at the top of an organization certainly control the purse strings and can decide what programs stay and what programs go. These people can effect change. But the individuals responsible for program delivery are those who will ultimately bring about change in a program. Whether it is carried out in a formal setting where the entire staff is present for the same slide presentation and receives the same written report, or whether it consists of informal, one-on-one discussions, the program providers must receive the evaluation results.

Once final evaluation results are made, the planning process begins anew. If results show that objectives were not met completely or not at all, changes are called for. Evaluation material collected throughout the program must be reviewed to help develop procedures for overcoming deficiencies or altering procedures in program presentation. If programs are successful and results exceed expectations, evaluation material can help identify why these programs were successful and, if possible, incorporate these elements into other programs.

Finally, the evaluation results can be used to determine the need for growth.

Does evidence indicate that programs can be expanded?

Does evidence exist that new programs are needed?

Were the occurrence of certain results an aberration that occurred only because of specific circumstances that are not in the control of the program providers?

Have new standards come into effect since program initiation, or are new standards on the horizon that will not be met based on the evaluation of current programs?

Acting on these and other questions is likely to determine the progress and success of the organization. And evaluation is what will make addressing and answering these questions possible.

Planning Exercise
Goal Development

Working in groups of three to five, follow these steps to complete a mini-planning sequence:

1.a. Be sure that each person in the group is pursuing the same exercise-related profession (for example, secondary school physical educator, athletic trainer at the college/university level, physical therapist in a sports medicine clinic, exercise specialist in a cardiac rehabilitation program).

1.b. Brainstorm to develop a list of goals you would like to accomplish as a professional in this area. Be creative. Don't limit yourself. Stop only when the group can come up with no more ideas.

1.c. Examine the list. Do you see things that you think are not likely to be accomplished in any program? If so, eliminate them.

1.d. Prioritize the remaining list. As a group, decide on the 10 things on the list that are most important to the professional area. If you have fewer than 10 items, simply rank-order the items with the most important being number 1. (In an actual planning situation, you would not limit your list. It is suggested here simply to speed the exercise.)

2.a. Obtain an outside source that contains guidelines for programs in the exercise-related professions. Examples of sources are:

>A State Physical Education Curriculum Guide
>AAHPERD's *Basic Stuff Series I and II*
>Athletic Training Program Guidelines from NATA
>Fitness Program Guidelines from ACSM
>*Healthy People 2000: Promoting Health/Preventing Disease: Objectives for the Nation*
>NCAA Guidelines for Athletic Program Compliance to Title IX.

2.b. Peruse the guidelines for goal statements, objectives, directives, mandates, and the like.

2.c. Compare your findings to your top 10 goals. Are you on target? If not, make the appropriate changes. If your group feels strongly about some things on the original list, do not replace them with items from the outside source. Simply add to your list any items from the outside source.

3.a. Examine your list closely. Does a common thread run through all the items, or do the items fall naturally into groups with each group having a common thread?

3.b. If one common thread emerges, develop a mission statement for your professional program that emphasizes that common thread and how you will accomplish the primary purpose of the program. If more than one major area of emphasis becomes apparent, develop a mission statement incorporating each major idea and describing how you will accomplish the primary purposes of your program. Make sure the mission statement includes your philosophy about the importance of your purpose.

You are now at the point at which you can quantify your primary purpose (goal) and begin to develop objectives that will guide your program and your evaluation.

Planning Exercise
Determining Methods of Evaluation

This is a continuation of the goal-setting exercise. Students who have not had an evaluation or test-and-measurement course might find this exercise challenging. It is included here as an indication of the preplanning necessary for evaluation. Financial and personnel resources are necessary to have an effective evaluation program, and the use of these resources must be planned in advance.

4.a. Look back at the list of goals in step 2.c of the goal development exercise. Consider the types of changes that will occur if these goals are accomplished. Make a list of changes expected.

4.b. Categorize the changes (put changes that have do with change in knowledge together, put changes that have to do with change in skill together, put changes that have to do with attitude together, and so on).

4.c. Consider the types of data needed to indicate the changes. For example, do you need pre- and post- information? Do you need demographic information? Do you need to test for knowledge? Do you need to assess attitudes?

4.d. Make a list of the methods of evaluation that can be used to gather the information you need for indicating change.

4.e. Determine how these evaluation tools can be obtained and what resources are needed to do so (for example, can these be purchased, can they be constructed in-house, what is the cost in dollars, in time, is the expertise available, and so on).

NOTES

1. C. A. Bucher, and M. L. Krotee, *Management of Physical Education and Sport*, 11th edition (Boston: WCB/McGraw-Hill, 1998).
2. Described by J. T. Butler, *Principles of Health Education and Health Promotion*, 2d edition (Englewood, CO: Morton Publishing, 1997).
3. J. F. McKenzie and J. L. Jurs, *Planning, Implementing, and Evaluating Health Promotion Programs, A Primer* (New York: Macmillan, 1993).
4. McKenzie and Jurs.
5. McKenzie and Jurs.
6. J. H. Railey and P. R. Tschauner, *Managing Physical Education, Fitness, and Sports Programs*, 2d edition (Mountain View, CA: Mayfield Publishing, 1993).

RESOURCES

American Alliance for Health, Physical Education, Recreation and Dance. (1987). *Basic Stuff Series, I and II.* Reston, VA: AAHPERD.

American Alliance for Health, Physical Education, Recreation and Dance. (1988). *Physical Best.* Reston, VA: AAHPERD.

American College of Sports Medicine. (1997). *Exercise Management for Persons with Chronic Diseases and Disabilities.* Champaign, IL: Human Kinetics.

American Public Health Association. (1991). *Healthy Communities 2000: Model Standards — Guidelines for Community Attainment of the Year 2000 National Health Objectives*, 3d ed. Washington, DC: APHA.

Arnheim, D. D., and W. E. Prentice, (1997). *Principles of Athletic Training*, 9th ed. St. Louis, MO: McGraw-Hill Co., Inc.

Baumgartner, T. A. (1987). *Measurement for Evaluation in Physical Education and Exercise Science*, 3d ed. Dubuque, IA: Wm. C. Brown Publishers.

Jubenville, A. (1993). *Outdoor Recreation and Management*, 3d ed. State College, PA: Venture Publishing.

Kestner, J. L. (1996). *Program Evaluation for Sport Directors* (American Sport Education Program). Champaign, IL: Human Kinetics.

Leith, L. M. (1990). *Coaches Guide to Sport Administration.* Champaign, IL: Leisure Press.

Mull, R. F. (1997). *Recreational Sport Management*, 3d ed. Champaign, IL: Human Kinetics.

National Association for Sport and Physical Education. (1995). *Moving into the Future: National Standards for Physical Education — A Guide to Content and Assessment.* St. Louis: Mosby Year Book.

National Association for Sport and Physical Education. (1995). *National Standards for Athletic Coaches.* Reston, VA: NASPE.

Pritchard, R. E. (1990). *Fitness, Inc.: A Guide to Corporate Health and Wellness Programs.* Homewood, IL: Dow Jones-Irwin Publishers.

Rankin, J. M. (1995). *Athletic Training Management: Concepts and Applications.* St. Louis: C. V. Mosby.

Ray, R. (1994). *Management Strategies in Athletic Training.* Champaign, IL: Human Kinetics.

Sullivan, J. V. (1990). *Management of Health and Fitness Programs.* Springfield, IL: Charles C. Thomas Publishers.

U. S. Department of Health and Human Services. (1989). *Promoting Health/Preventing Disease: Year 2000 Objectives for the Nation.* Washington, DC: U. S. Government Printing Office.

Introduction to the Law

OBJECTIVES

After studying this chapter, you should be able to:

1. Define common law and discuss the role of precedent in establishing common law.
2. List and discuss the subsystems that make up our system of law.
3. Differentiate civil and criminal law.
4. Describe the steps followed in a criminal law suit.

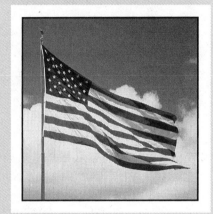

For some time, a basic understanding of legal foundations has been included in the preparation for students in exercise-related professions. When exercise-related professionals were considered to be primarily physical education teachers and athletic coaches, the legal concerns centered on teachers' and coaches' duty to their students and athletes and, more specifically, to the breach of this duty, or *negligence*, by the teacher or coach. Even though negligence is still an important concern to exercise professionals, they now have to be familiar with many more legal concepts.

This change has resulted from both the increases in variety of vocations available to exercise professionals and to the introduction of both old and new legal concepts into the exercise field. For example, negligence is considered not only in school settings, where teachers or coaches have a well-established duty to their minor charges, but also to the cardiac rehabilitation center, or the industrial wellness center, or the local fitness center, where the clients are more likely to be adults and where standards of professional care may reach higher levels.

Also, discrimination now is not likely to be related only to Title IX concerns in athletic programs or physical education classes but also to sexual harassment claims under the 1964 Civil Rights Act in virtually any setting where exercise professionals might find themselves employed.

Because of the growing numbers of legal issues with which exercise professionals have to be familiar, they must first have a general understanding of the law and legal concepts. This helps answer some of the "why" questions they might have concerning application of the law to specific situations and also shows the relationship between laws.

THE BASIC STRUCTURE OF U. S. LEGAL SYSTEM

The law of the United States is derived from both the *common law*, including precedent, and *statutory law*.

Common Law

Common law

Common law is the system of law derived from custom and precedent. Founders of this country brought with them the common law of England developed through *custom* and used it as the basis for law in the United States. The common law grew out of a desire to have some system that would help manage the relationships between people.

For example, one of the oldest forms of common law is the law of trespass. The law of trespass came about so a person who was trespassed against could collect damages against the trespasser — be it for trespassing against one's person or against one's property. Since one's person and one's property were held in high regard in early England, it was reasonable to expect that if any person caused damage to person or property, that person should pay (in some way) for the damage. Today, we still hold our person and property in high regard, and we still adhere to laws of trespass that have been passed down to us over time through custom.

Precedent

Precedent

Laws based on *precedent* also are derived from what has transpired over time. Precedent, however, refers specifically to a court decision that continues to be followed as an example of how specific laws should be interpreted. In the United States today, we still follow the decisions of courts in early England, especially in the area of property ownership.

When laws were written to establish the passage of ownership from a father to his offspring, the courts often were asked to interpret those laws and make decisions as to which offspring would receive what property under the law. If the court decided that the law was to be interpreted to mean that the eldest son should receive 50% of the estate and all children shared the remainder equally, one precedent was set. On the other hand, if the court decided that all children should receive equal shares of the estate regardless of age or sex, another precedent was set.

Once set, precedent may be carried on for an indeterminate time. Or precedent may be broken when a later court decides that an earlier court was wrong or that what a court decided earlier is no longer applicable in today's world and should be changed — thereby establishing a new precedent.

Courts that set precedent are usually judging a case that is being appealed from a lower court decision. Any court decision can be precedent-setting; however, those on appeal tend to be more far-reaching. Appeals are brought when one (or both, in some instances) of the parties in the case has reason to believe that there was an error in the conduct of the case or an error in rendering the judgment. The party appeals the case to a higher court in the hope that the higher court will find fault with the lower court decision and give a different ruling. The higher the level of the court hearing the appeal, the more influence its decisions will have concerning setting precedent.

In the United States, the U.S. Supreme Court is the highest court to hear appeals and would have the greatest influence on precedent in the areas of law it has considered. If the U.S. Supreme Court has made no decisions in a given area of the law, however, a Federal Court of Appeals or Federal District Court may be the court that has set precedent in a given area. When this is the case, the decision of the Court of Appeals or District Court establishes precedent for its geographical region only and not any other regions. Courts in other regions may follow the precedent of another Court of Appeals or District Court if they so wish.

Even though precedent may vary in any one area of the law from region to region, it will not vary radically. If it does, the U.S. Supreme Court will take a case involving that area of law and settle the variance by handing down a decision, which then becomes precedent for all regions.

The same process is followed at the state level, where the state's highest court establishes precedent for the rest of the state when it hands down a decision on a particular law. As long as the high court has not made a decision on an area of the law, the decisions of lower state courts may set precedent. What is precedent in one state may not be precedent in another state. In many cases, state courts that are considering a law for the first time will look to decisions from courts in other states (particularly those in their own district) to see how that issue was decided

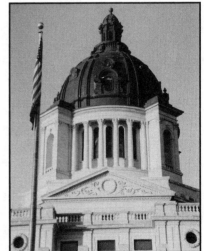

State Capitol building.

there. Even then, the state court may decide to go its own way and not follow the precedent of another state.

Precedent is most often connected to fairness and justice within the legal system. Because other courts have decided cases with a certain set of circumstances in a given way, it would seem only fair to those in cases with similar circumstances for their cases to be decided in the same manner now and in the future. If you were to live in South Carolina and were involved in a case in which you were facing a claim of negligence, you would expect that the facts in your case would be treated no different from someone involved in the same type of case in New York, and certainly no different from one in North Carolina. You would expect precedent to be followed. If your case were to have some special circumstances, however, you would expect justice to be done whether that would mean following precedent or setting a new precedent. Either way, precedent would work to ensure the correct outcome in the case.

Precedent also is important in helping someone understand how to act in his or her profession. When precedent is set in a case where a professional has been judged as negligent in meeting his or her duty to a participant in an activity program, we learn that whatever standard of care the negligent party was providing was not sufficient. Over time, precedent paints a descriptive picture of what we must do in our profession to meet our standard of care to those who participate in our programs.

Statutory Law

Statutory law

In addition to common law and precedent, laws are established by statute. *Statutes* are laws passed at the various levels of government to control the behavior of the citizenry. The federal government passes laws dealing with national issues. States, counties, and municipalities pass laws dealing with state and local issues. These governmental bodies also formulate regulations that have to do with applying laws and with running agencies that provide services to the citizenry. These regulations often have the effect of law because the courts consider the regulations when the laws related to the regulations are broken. Therefore, following the regulations as if they were laws is wise. Most exercise-related professionals have little difficulty stating the "one-sentence law" on equal opportunity in educational programs that receive federal funds, known as Title IX. Few, however, will ever know the intricacies of the many regulations that determine areas covered by Title IX and how these regulations are met and enforced. Through the regulations, persons responsible for meeting Title IX's mandate are held accountable.

Common law and *statutory law* are interconnected. Statutory laws are often written to reinforce common law. Even as trespass on one's person is an ancient common law, it is also reflected in our statutory laws of murder, manslaughter, sexual assault, battery, and so forth. Likewise, statutes against robbery, burglary, larceny, and the like reinforce the common law of trespass against one's property.

When courts hear cases dealing with statutory laws, they hand down decisions that may be appealed. Decisions of the appellate courts establish precedent, which then becomes common law as to how that law is dealt with based on circumstances in that particular case.

The U.S. system of law can be defined as four separate but interrelated subsystems:[1]

1. A system for defining relationships between people
2. A system of principles that tell us how to behave
3. A system for establishing reasonableness in our behavior, and
4. A system that creates and limits freedom.

Exercise-related professionals will enter the workforce in a people-oriented profession. Their professional life will be one of relationships — with the student, the athlete, the patient, the employee, the club member, and so on. This relationship will be one primarily of duty owed to someone seeking a service. The service might be education, or therapy, or exercise instruction. Laws concerning liability and negligence will affect this relationship. Laws concerning contracts also can enter the relationship — not only the relationship with the client but also the relationship with employers and co-workers.

When the law is considered as a system of principles that tell us how to behave and as a method of establishing reasonableness within our behavior, the exercise professional should realize that the relationship is still what is being considered. Only now it is specific behavior that is typically targeted by a law or laws. Behavior such as unwanted sexual attention that can be interpreted as sexual harassment is an example. Other examples are unwanted touching that can be viewed as sexual harassment or battery, and conversation to one party about a third party that can be viewed as slander.

When the law is viewed as a system that both creates and limits freedom, the rights created by the Constitution of the United States are being considered. The Constitution grants rights such as freedom of speech, freedom to assemble, freedom from unwarranted search and seizure, the right to due process under the law, the right to equal protection under the law, and the right to privacy, among others. The federal government and state governments (through the Fourteenth Amendment) cannot pass any laws that abridge these rights without an overriding state purpose. Abridgement of these rights, however, does not stop with governmental entities, because the federal government has passed laws ensuring that individuals and private entities do not violate these special rights. Laws that protect against discrimination based on race, gender, disability, and age have the primary purpose of protecting our right to due process and equal protection, and are applicable to nearly anyone who would attempt to violate these rights.

The exercise-related professional working in a governmental agency such as a public school, college/university, or hospital should be particularly cognizant of this facet of the law. Those working in large corporations and in any business that meets the criteria to which these laws are directed must also be aware of these laws and how the laws might impact on them in their profession.

CRIMINAL VERSUS CIVIL LAW

Criminal (penal) law

If a professional violates a law in any of the systems named above, he or she could face criminal or civil charges. Criminal charges could be brought by violating the *penal law* of the United States or of any individual state, municipality, or other governmental entity. Penal laws are those for which the violator is expected to make some satisfaction to the public. Some governmental entity — the United States, an individual state, municipality, or other entity — will bring charges against the violator on behalf of the public. The individual may violate the penal law by doing something that is prohibited or by failing to do something that is required.

Examples to which we can all relate are the laws associated with highway and vehicular safety. The public, through its representatives, has decided that drivers should not exceed certain speeds on the highways. The public also has decided that, while driving a vehicle on highways, individuals in the front seat should wear seatbelts. If you violate the speeding laws by driving too fast, you may be stopped and given a citation, for which you most likely will pay a fine or even serve time in jail. You have done something that the public has prohibited, and you will satisfy the public by paying a certain amount of money or being confined in jail. Likewise, if you are not wearing your seatbelt when you are stopped for speeding, you will be charged for failing to do something the public has said you should do, and you will satisfy the public for this also.

As a professional in a people-oriented profession, you might well be charged with violating a criminal, or penal, law. An exercise-related professional is often required to touch his or her clients. If a client perceives this touching as unwarranted and offensive, the client may bring criminal charges of battery or even sexual assault, depending on the nature of the touching. This will be examined in more detail later.

Even though the exercise-related professionals might find themselves facing criminal charges in relation to their professional duties, they are more likely to have civil actions brought against them. When civil law is violated, the violator has abridged the private rights of an individual or group of individuals. *Civil actions* are all actions that are not considered criminal. When we violate someone's private rights, that individual or group of individuals whose rights have been violated will bring an action against us, rather than the state, as is the case in a criminal action.   *Civil law*

An individual's private rights can be violated in a number of ways. These rights might be violated by being negligent in one's duty of care to someone participating in an activity program that results in an injury to that person. Even if the negligence is unintentional, the damage has been done, the right has been violated, and the person responsible for the injury is liable. A person's rights also might be violated intentionally. That person might be touched inappropriately, or have something untrue said about him that damages his reputation, or be held against his will, or he might have a contractual right violated.

An individual might be discriminated against because of race, color, creed, national origin, sex, age, or disability. An individual might not be given due process in an action that terminates her employment, or she might not receive equal protection under the law. An individual might be searched by an employer or be required to take a drug test in which the right against illegal search and seizure is violated. Each of these ways of violating an individual's private rights will be examined in chapters that follow.

ANATOMY OF A LAWSUIT

Regardless of how individuals' rights might be violated, they will follow the same procedure in bringing a claim against the person, or persons, they believe is responsible for the violation. First, the injured party, the *plaintiff*, files a claim, in the appropriate court, alleging that someone has violated a specific individual right. The plaintiff will state how the right was or is being violated. The plaintiff also will state the actions he is seeking to enforce, redress, or protect his particular right.   *Plaintiff*

The court now will give notice to the person(s) named in the claim that such a claim has been filed against him. The violator, the *defendant*, then is required to file an answer in the court. The court will review the claim and the answer to determine whether a case does indeed exist. Additional information might be requested from both parties.   *Defendant*

If you are wondering about the value of being aware of the anatomy of a lawsuit, there is no better place than here to mention that value. The exercise-related professional will continuously be required to keep records. Whether that professional is a teacher, coach, athletic trainer, therapist, fitness leader, or recreational specialist, she will be writing goals and objectives, plans for daily activities, periodic reports, accident reports, reports on participant progress, reports on maintenance and safety checks, and so on. These reports contain information about what the professional has done or has not done. These reports will show how the professional accepts and acts on the responsibilities of the job. These reports show the professional's patterns of behavior. If these reports exist and show the acceptance and completion of duties through active, positive patterns of behavior, the professional will have information, when requested, that supports her doing her duty. When these reports are not present, their absence indicates a pattern of not doing one's duty. Knowing ahead of time the importance of these reports as a paper trail makes a person more likely to complete and file these reports that so often are seen as an unnecessary part of one's job.

Settlement

Once all information is examined and the court has determined that a case exists, the court will seek to have the parties reach an agreement, a *settlement*, before going to trial. If no agreement can be reached, the lawsuit will move forward. The defendant has the right to have the case heard before a jury but can waive this right if he wishes. In such instances, the case then is heard before a judge only. In a civil case, the plaintiff has the burden of proving the defendant was the cause of the violation of her rights. This is done by proving the elements of the specific violation.

The most common violation brought against exercise-related professionals is negligence. The plaintiff must prove the elements of negligence against the defendant. These elements are duty, breach of duty, actual injury, and proximate cause. If the plaintiff fails to present evidence sufficient to prove each of these elements, the defendant will move for summary judgment following completion of the plaintiff's case. If the judge agrees that the elements have not been proven, summary judgment in favor of the defendant will be granted and the case will be over.

If the judge does not agree, the request for summary judgment will be denied and the case will continue. It is now the defendant's turn to present his case. He, too, must address the elements of the alleged violation. His purpose is to disprove what the plaintiff has presented by presenting evidence that supports his case.

Trier of fact
Preponderance
of the evidence

Once both sides have presented their cases and made their closings, the judge will make a decision in non-jury cases or send the case to the jury. In a jury trial, the judge gives the jury instructions on the law related to the case it must now decide before the jury begins to deliberate. The jury, the *trier of fact*, must decide whether the plaintiff has met her burden of proof by a *preponderance of the evidence* (more than 50%). This means that the jury thinks the weight of the evidence is in the plaintiff's favor. If it believes she has met this burden, they will find in her favor. If it thinks she has not met his burden, it will find for the defendant.

Once a decision has been reached, the jury will present the decision in court. If the decision is in the favor of the plaintiff, the decision will contain what the defendant must do to compensate the plaintiff for violating her rights. In the case of a negligence suit, the defendant would be responsible for paying actual, and possibly speculative, losses the plaintiff incurred. In certain cases the defendant might also have to pay punitive damages. In other civil cases, the defendant may have to reinstate a plaintiff employee with back pay or pay damages for loss of one's good name in a defamation case.

After the decision has been announced, either the plaintiff or the defendant may appeal the decision. An appeal, however, must be based on a presumed error in the conduct of the trial. Neither side can appeal simply because it did not like the outcome. The party that appeals does so because she believes the judge, the *trier of the law*, has made an error in conducting the trial. The appeal is made to a higher court in the jurisdiction in which the initial trial was held. If the appellate court decides to take the appeal, the party making the appeal has the burden to show that an error was made that affected the outcome of the case. The appellate court can uphold the lower court's decision, reverse the decision, or remand (send back) the case to the lower court for a new trial (after indicating a determined error).

Trier of the law

Once a decision is made concerning a case, whether in the initial trial or on appeal, the decision becomes part of precedent. Precedent is important because it determines how future cases with the same set of facts might be determined and also because it shows what we as a society expect in the relationships we have with one another. If we do not meet these expectations in the conduct of our professional and personal lives, we will be held accountable based on our laws and customs as established over time.

RECAP

Legal issues for exercise-related professionals have expanded because of the growth of the profession and because of the introduction of new legal concepts in the profession. No longer is the profession made up only of physical education teachers and coaches. It now reaches into corporate wellness centers and therapy clinics, as well as into new areas within the former settings — athletic training and sport management. No longer are we concerned only about negligence and disparate treatment of athletes under Title IX. Now we must be aware of sexual harassment and unwanted searches and seizures. We also must be more aware of due process and equal protection under the law and of potential violation of contractual rights.

Exercise-related professionals should be familiar with the bases of our legal system to better understand how the law affects their duties as professionals as the law is interpreted in today's courts. Our laws are a system of laws based on common law arrived at through custom and precedent and on statutes passed by our federal, state, and local governments. How the courts deal with these laws sets precedent for how the laws will be viewed in the future. The precedent also might determine the passage of new laws. The higher the court setting the precedent, the more influence it has on the law.

The law can be viewed as several sets of systems — systems that define our relationships with others, establish behavior, establish reasonableness in behavior, and create and limit freedoms. The precedent set in our courts in relation to these systems influences not only the law but also the conduct of those who must follow the law as they interact with others.

If we violate laws within these systems, we will likely face civil or criminal charges. If we are charged criminally, we will be tried by the state on behalf of the victim and the public in general. If we are charged civilly, the victim will take us to court. In either case, we will stand as a defendant against a plaintiff state or an individual victim. In the exercise-related professions, one could violate the state's criminal laws, but more likely one will violate an individual's private rights, resulting in civil charges. This would involve going through the process of a civil trial. The plaintiff victim would attempt to prove the elements of the alleged violation while the defendant would attempt to counter the claim. Regardless of who wins, the outcome will become part of the precedent of future cases.

Exercise-related professionals who are aware of the law as it relates to their profession are more likely to know how to conduct themselves in their profession. They are more likely not to find themselves in court to begin with, but if they do, they are more likely to be part of precedent that shows what should be done rather than what should not be done as a professional.

NOTES

1. L. J. Carpenter, *Legal Concepts in Sport: A Primer* (Reston, VA: American Alliance for Health, Physical Education, Recreation, and Dance, 1995).

RESOURCES

Dougherty, N. J. et al. (1994). *Sport, Physical Activity, and the Law.* Champaign, IL: Human Kinetics Publishers.

Nolan, J. R., and J. M. Nolan-Haley. (1990). *Black's Law Dictionary*, 6th ed. St. Paul: West Publishing.

Tort Law

OBJECTIVES

After studying this chapter, you should be able to:

1. Define and give an example of a tort.
2. Discuss the reasons for increases in civil lawsuits in our society.
3. Describe the concept of fault and relate it to the establishment of liability.
4. Be able to define the following terms of tort law: liability, negligence, damages, duty, breach, proximate cause.
5. Distinguish between an unintentional and an intentional tort.
6. Discuss the four elements of negligence.
7. Differentiate gross negligence and negligence.
8. Give four methods used to counter claims of negligence.
9. Describe the difference between contributory and comparative negligence and give the rationale for moving away from the practice of contributory negligence to comparative negligence.
10. List the general elements of an intentional tort and give three examples of an intentional tort with the specific elements of each example.
11. Give examples of ways in which exercise-related professionals could commit an unintentional or intentional tort, and suggest how to avoid the tort.

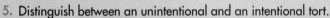

A *tort* is a wrong committed upon the person or property of one person by another, typically resulting in injury to the wronged person or his property. The person committing the wrong is the *tort-feasor*, and the wronged person is the injured party. Tort law is that area of the law that deals with remedying wrongs that one person

Tort

Tort-feasor

does to another. The wrong by the tort-feasor can be of a criminal or a civil nature. If the wrong is criminal, the state will bring charges against the tort-feasor on behalf of the injured party, the victim, and society in general. If the wrong is civil, the injured party must bring action by filing a claim against the tort-feasor in court. Even if the tort is criminal, there may also be a civil component to the injury that the injured party might take to court.

We have to look no further than the infamous O. J. Simpson trials, in which Mr. Simpson was tried in criminal court by the state for murder and then taken to civil court by the parents of one of the murdered victims for the victim's wrongful death. He was found not guilty beyond a reasonable doubt for the murder but was found liable for the wrongful death of the victim and was required to compensate the injured party (the parents) for that injury.

Although exercise-related professionals are not exempt from criminal torts, they are much more likely to be involved in a civil suit brought by the injured party. You have no doubt heard the statement, "We live in a suit-happy society." Whether we do or do not is open to debate. In any event, there has been a noticeable increase in civil lawsuits brought against alleged tort-feasors in U. S. courts in recent years. Possible reasons for the increase in cases where wronged persons are seeking a remedy are: (1) insurance shortfalls, (2) the right to sue, (3) the doctrine of entitlement, (4) settlements, and (5) the myth of being risk-free.[1]

1. *Insurance shortfalls* no doubt play a major role in the increase of civil tort cases. If an individual is injured and her insurance pays for only a portion of the costs of this injury, the individual must pay out of her own pocket the costs the insurance does not cover. If the individual believes someone else was either totally or partially responsible for the injury, she believes the tort-feasor should bear part or all of the costs and that she, the injured party, should not be responsible for those costs. Claims are made, and a lawsuit ensues.

2. People are more likely to be aware of their *right to sue* today and are freer to make use of that right. Our civil law system has always provided the means for remedies for injury to our persons or property even though these might have been limited in some way. For example, if the government (or someone acting on behalf of the government) caused the injury, the injured party could not expect to receive any compensation from the government because of the *doctrine of sovereign immunity*. This doctrine prohibited bringing suit against the government without its permission — and the government rarely gave its permission to be sued. The federal government has now waived its immunity to suits by law, and most states have done the same through state laws for state and local governments.

Doctrine of sovereign immunity

Another limiting factor to using the legal system to help restore losses from injury was the practice by the tort-feasor of using *contributory negligence* as a defense against liability for an injury. Under this practice, if the tort-feasor could prove that the injured party had in any way contributed to the injury by his own negligence, all of the liability could be transferred to the injured party and the tort-feasor would have no liability.

Contributory negligence

The inequity of this legal practice was finally realized, and today this practice has been replaced by one of *comparative negligence*. Under the practice of comparative negligence, both the injured party and the tort-feasor are responsible for whatever portion of the injury that each caused (with some exceptions that will be discussed later). With the removal of these two stumbling blocks, the injured party is apt to believe that suits are more likely to result in a favorable outcome for him. Add to this less respect for those in higher positions, and it is understandable that individuals who have experienced an injury will take advantage of their right to sue.

Comparative negligence

3. Adding to the feeling of a more favorable outcome by the injured party is the *doctrine of entitlement*. This is not an actual legal doctrine but, rather, a phenomenon associated with our jury system. When an injured party brings her case to court, she often is viewed sympathetically by the jury, which believes that someone must pay. This is especially true when children or elderly people are the injured parties. This is also true when the "little person" or the "common person" goes up against a giant corporation or the government as the alleged tort-feasor. The jury, acting in humanitarian fashion, is likely to think that providing compensation to the injured party is a responsibility that it must meet, especially since the jury thinks the tort-feasor is more than able to pay.

Doctrine of entitlement

4. Injured parties are not the only ones who know that juries may be swayed by presentation of information dealing with the pain and suffering of the injured party. Those who are named in the suit as the person or entity responsible for the pain and suffering know this also. Because of this, *settlements* out of court are likely. The vast majority of civil tort cases (an estimated 85%) never go to court because they are settled out of court. Of course, a case can never be settled if it is not brought. Whether the injured party is anticipating a settlement out of court or a win before a jury, he has sufficient reason to believe that he will receive some compensation for his injuries and is therefore encouraged to sue.

5. The above reasons for increased likelihood of suing are magnified in the area of exercise-related professions when the nature of the profession is considered. Most of the exercise-related professions involve activities that are risky, whether it is exercise for an employee in a corporate wellness program or a contact sport at the professional level. The *myth of being risk-free* is just that — a myth — and this myth is twofold.

First, individuals participating in the activities that exercise-related professionals offer expect the activities to be safe and do not do everything they can to prevent an injury. When they are injured, they are angered and likely are to sue even if they are responsible, totally or in part, for the injury.

The second aspect of this myth is that the professional does not recognize and fully appreciate the participant's lack of understanding of the risks. Therefore, they do not assure that participants fully understand the risks. When a participant is injured, the lack of full disclosure of possible risks and any lack of instruction, prior to beginning the activity, in ways to avoid the risks, adds fuel to the fire and increases the likelihood that the injured participant will sue.

THE CONCEPT OF FAULT

Fault

No matter what the motivation for the increasing number of tort lawsuits in U. S. society, we as a society believe that when someone is harmed by the actions of another, that individual has the right to seek a remedy for the injury. To determine who should be responsible for returning this person to her pre-injury state, we have developed the concept of *fault*. Fault is an error or defect of judgment or of conduct by one who is responsible for the safety of others in her care. Fault results from inattention, incapacity, or perversity.

Liability

Vicarious liability

Fault also acknowledges relationships between persons when more than one person might be responsible for an injury. Employers, or their businesses in general, can be held liable for the acts of their employees. This is known as *vicarious liability*. Vicarious liability can be either *personal* or *institutional*. In vicarious liability that is personal, the employer is liable for the acts of employees because of negligent hiring, negligent retention, lack of supervision, lack of adequate training, and the like. In vicarious liability that is institutional, the business or institution is liable for the acts of its employees because the employee is the *agent* acting for the business.

When someone is found to be at fault for the injury of another (whether it is an individual or a business), we have decided that the responsible party should compensate the injured party. Typically, paying for the procedures necessary to make the person whole again or to put that person back as near as possible to where he would have been had the injury not occurred does this.

Damages

The person seeking to be made whole again would seek *damages* from the tort-feasor. These damages might be *actual* (or *compensatory*), *speculative*, or *punitive*.

Actual damages are those directly related to an injury. These include any hospital or rehabilitation costs the injured party expends to recover from the injury. If the injured party was employed at the time of injury, actual damages also would include lost wages or the value of lost or decreased productivity.

Actual damages

In addition to actual damages, the injured party may seek speculative damages, such as loss of future wages or production. If the injured party will never return to work or never will become a superstar athlete because of the injury, she will speculate what the losses will be over her expected career and seek those damages. Third parties related to the injured party may also bring speculative damages against the tort-feasor. Loss of love and affection and loss of consortium (conjugal relations between husband and wife) are the most typical third-party damages brought. These third-party damages are typically sought in extreme cases in which the injured party has died or the injury is severe enough to prevent normal functioning of the injured party, such as partial or total paralysis.

Speculative damages

The injured party may also seek punitive damages against the tort-feasor. As a society, we have decided that in addition to making an injured person whole, the injured person should be able to "punish" the tort-feasor. The purpose of the punishment is to increase the chances that the tort-feasor will not commit the same tort again. The punishment also has the purpose of sending a message to others that this type of behavior will not be tolerated and they, too, will be punished in the same manner if they commit such a tort. When seeking punitive damages, the injured party must show that the tort-feasor acted willfully, maliciously, or fraudulently. In most states, the injured party presents a claim of gross negligence against the tort-feasor when seeking punitive damages. (Negligence and gross negligence are discussed in more detail later.)

Punitive damages

Fault may be *intentional* or *unintentional*. When fault is intentional, we think in terms of criminal acts of the person at fault and typically seek recompense through the state in a criminal trial. When fault is unintentional, we think in terms of *negligence* and seek recompense in a civil action brought by the injured party. Although the exercise-related professional is not immune to intentional torts of a criminal nature, he will most likely face unintentional torts of a civil nature on a day-to-day basis.

UNINTENTIONAL TORTS

Unintentional tort

Students who are preparing to be exercise-related professionals commonly reject the concept of fault, particularly in the area of unintentional torts. They reason that if the professional did not mean to harm the participant and the participant freely chose to be involved in the activity, how can the professional be held responsible for the injury? This reasoning ignores our expectations of reasonable persons who are in charge of the activities they offer.

The law of *negligence* is founded on reasonable conduct by reasonable persons in any given situation. When a person fails to use such care as a reasonably prudent and careful person would use under similar circumstances and the person to whom they owe this duty of care is injured, the person who owed the care is at fault — even when the lack of care was unintentional. Society has determined that you must act as a reasonable person, and when you do not, you are held liable for any resulting injury and the losses the victim suffers as a result of the injury.

Proving Negligence

Negligence

Being in a position of care does not automatically result in one's being at fault (negligent) when someone in that person's care is injured. The injury might be purely accidental — something over which no one had control — or the injury might not have been related in any way to the duty of care owed by the person in charge. If there is an injury, injured parties have several alternatives at their disposal depending upon the cause of the injury.

- They can accept responsibility for the injury and bear the liability for any loss associated with the injury alone.

- They can seek and receive compensation from the person in whose care they were at the time of the injury (without ever filing a case against that person).

- If they seek compensation and the person from whom they seek compensation claims no liability, the injured party can file a lawsuit and take the alleged tort-feasor to court.

In the latter case, if the court decides there are sufficient grounds for the claim, the suit will go forward. If the two parties cannot reach a settlement out of court, the suit will go to trial, where the injured party becomes the plaintiff who must present sufficient evidence to convince a jury that the *preponderance of the evidence* (more than 50%) is against the alleged tort-feasor (the defendant). To do this, she must prove the elements of negligence: duty, breach of duty, injury, and proximate cause.

1. *Duty.* In the exercise-related professions, duty to participants is typically indisputable. Duty arises as a result of the nature of the relationship between the participant and the person in control of the activity in which the participant is involved. Teachers, coaches, and athletic trainers are clearly responsible for the care and safety of their students and athletes while in their charge, especially when these students and athletes are minors. Recreational personnel are responsible for the care and safety of participants in a wide range of activities. Fitness and wellness personnel are responsible for clients in activities ranging from weight-loss programs to cardiac rehabilitation. Therapists are responsible for the safety and care of their patients when administering the various protocols used in rehabilitation. *[Duty]*

What the plaintiff must show is that the injury sustained did indeed occur while she was participating in the activity in which the alleged defendant's duty arises. The defendant, of course, will attempt to show, if applicable, that the plaintiff's injury was caused by some act of the plaintiff that was in no way related to the activity in which the defendant owed the plaintiff a duty of care (see discussion below).

2. *Breach of duty.* In addition to establishing a duty of care by the defendant, the plaintiff must show that the defendant breached the duty. This breach is what is at the heart of the claim of negligence. In a claim of negligence, the plaintiff is concerned primarily with showing that the defendant unintentionally did something a reasonably prudent professional would not have done. The defendant might have unintentionally omitted something in the procedure that should have followed, called *omission*. The defendant might have unintentionally committed an error by adding something that was not necessary in the procedure, called *commission*. Regardless as to whether the breach was the result of omission or commission, the plaintiff will win if he can show that such breach did indeed occur and resulted in the next two elements of negligence. *[Breach of duty]* *[Omission]* *[Commission]*

3. *Injury.* The elements of injury and proximate cause are closely related and are generally considered together. People in exercise-related professions might breach their duty more than they would like to admit. Someone forgets to perform a regularly scheduled maintenance check on time. A playing field is not checked for hazards before a class or a game. A player is inserted into a game to play a position for which she has not received adequate training. As luck would have it, though, no one is injured and there is no negligence suit because no one was harmed.

At other times individuals participating in exercise-related programs are injured and no one is at fault. The injury is truly the result of an unfortunate series of circumstances over which no one had control and is one no one could have foreseen. The plaintiff has the burden to show that an actual injury has occurred and that the breach of duty by the defendant was the proximate, or direct, cause of the resulting injury, and not merely an accident. To prove injury, the plaintiff must show that he has suffered some damage or loss. This entails showing physical damage to one's person or property or some loss that may be strictly monetary or personal (as in loss of reputation). It may also involve a combination of these, wherein the plaintiff has suffered a physical injury that results in the loss of ability to perform. If the plaintiff's injury is not obvious or easily ascertained, the defendant will attempt to show that no injury exists and the plaintiff has incurred no actual loss.

Proximate cause

4. *Proximate cause.* Even if the plaintiff is successful in presenting evidence of an actual injury, she must prove that the defendant's breach of duty was the direct cause of the injury. It is not improbable that an individual who has been injured through no one's fault other than her own or through a completely uncontrollable set of circumstances will try to put the liability for the injury on someone other than herself or fate. To show proximate cause, the plaintiff must prove that there was a continuous sequence of events from the breach of duty to her actual injury; no intervening events could have caused the injury other than the breach; except for the breach, no injury would have been incurred.

Gross Negligence

A plaintiff seeking compensation from a defendant because of negligence might be seeking more than actual damages. He also may be seeking punitive damages as a means of punishing the defendant for his action or lack of action. Most jurisdictions require that actual losses be sustained before the plaintiff can seek punitive damages.

Gross negligence

In addition to proving actual losses, most jurisdictions require the plaintiff to prove something more than basic negligence. The negligence must rise to a level that would indicate wanton or intentional disregard for the safety of others. This is typically known as *gross negligence*.

Gross negligence must not be confused with an intentional tort. The "intent" of gross negligence is the intentional neglect of one's duty. It is an "I don't care" attitude that indicates a lack of concern for others' safety. The intent falls short of an intentional act to cause harm to someone through a specific action or inaction.

Exercise-related professionals should be careful not to establish patterns that might be interpreted as a lack of concern for the safety of others. A professional might continuously fail to perform regular safety inspections but no one is ever injured. When someone is injured, this past history of neglect might be all that is needed to show wanton disregard for the safety of others even though the problem was one of forgetfulness and not intent. Doing one's duty is the best defense against negligence, or against gross negligence.

Countering Claims of Negligence

The following information is typically presented in legal texts as "defenses against negligence." This is a misleading term. The only true defense against negligence is diligence on the part of professionals to meet their duty of care to persons participating in their programs. (Meeting the standard of care is discussed in Chapter 16 under risk management.) With that said, the following strategies might be used to show that the professional was not at fault or to reduce liability if at fault:

1. *Contributory/comparative negligence.* The defendant in a negligence case may attempt to prove that the injured party failed to meet the duty of protecting herself and was therefore injured as a result of her own *contributory negligence.* Because the plaintiff did not act as a reasonable person would be expected to act, she is at fault. This is considered an affirmative defense — one in which the defendant is attempting to show that he is in no way negligent and, therefore, is not liable for the defendant's injuries. The defendant may use this defense even in cases where he was negligent but the negligence had nothing to do with the injury suffered by the plaintiff. If a jury is convinced by the defendant's evidence that the plaintiff was totally responsible for her own injury, the defendant would owe no compensation to the plaintiff.

Under the newer practice of *comparative negligence*, a defendant who is negligent would still use contributory negligence by the plaintiff to reduce his liability, and in some cases to escape liability altogether. Under a *modified comparative negligence* plan, some states have a *threshold* for the plaintiff's liability that, if exceeded, bars recovery from the defendant. The threshold is typically 50%–51%. For instance, if the case takes place in a state that has a 51% threshold and the plaintiff and the defendant are found to be equally liable (50/50) for the injury, the plaintiff would be responsible for 50% of the proven damages. If the plaintiff were found to be 51% responsible for the injury, however, the defendant would owe the plaintiff nothing.

This threshold policy is closely related to the contributory negligence policy of the past, in which the defendant could be totally exonerated of any liability (even when liable) if the plaintiff was liable to any degree. For some time, the general legal practice was to consider that, because the injured party was at fault, the defendant should not be held liable to any degree. The trend in most states today is not to let defendants escape liability if their negligence did indeed contribute to the plaintiff's injury in some way.

Most states have moved to a policy of *pure comparative negligence*. Only a few states follow the policy of establishing a threshold above which the tort-feasor is totally exonerated. In pure comparative negligence states, the plaintiff must still prove the elements of negligence against the defendant to establish liability. The defendant will counter by attempting to establish contributory negligence, either partially or totally, by the plaintiff. The judge then directs the jury to consider whether either side was or was not negligent. If the jury finds both sides negligent to some degree, the jury must decide to what degree each party was negligent and assign liability accordingly. If the jury finds the defendant 15% liable, the defendant will be responsible for paying 15% of the plaintiff's proven damages. If the jury finds the defendant 85% liable, the defendant will be responsible for paying 85% of the plaintiff's proven damages.

Some legal advisors have noted that, if the defense does not use contributory or comparative negligence as part of its case and simply bases the case on not being negligent, the judge is barred from giving instructions on comparative negligence. This then puts the onus on the members of the jury to be aware of their state's laws concerning comparative negligence and to decide the case accordingly. The defense, of course, depends on the jury members not being familiar with those laws and deciding the case on the old contributory negligence standard where assumption of risk exonerated the tort-feasor. This may not seem just, but it is legal.

Assumption of the risks

2. *Assumption of risks*. Whereas the defense of contributory negligence depends on the lack of reasonableness and fault of the participant/plaintiff, the defense of assumption of the risks depends on consent and voluntariness of the participant/plaintiff. Under a defense of contributory negligence, the defendant would seek to totally escape liability (in threshold states where the plaintiff's fault exceeded the defendant's fault) or to reduce his liability (in pure comparative negligence states). Using a defense of assumption of the risks, the defendant is seeking to escape liability by showing that the injury the plaintiff suffered was attributable to the inherent risks of the activity, not the defendant's negligence.

Consent by the participant may be express, or it may be implied. *Express consent* is given by signing a *waiver* or *release* in which the participant accepts the risks of the activity and waives or releases the persons in charge of the activity from any liability for injuries that occur as a result of the nature of the activity. Express consent may also be given in *participation agreements,* in which the participant recognizes the inherent risks of the activity and takes responsibility for protecting herself (but does not release the persons in charge of liability). Parents commonly give consent for participants who are minors.

Implied consent is no less real than express consent, but there is nothing in writing. Implied consent is shown by the participant's willingness to participate in an activity even though risks are present. The classic case here is the person who attends a baseball game and chooses to sit in a nonscreened area of the ballpark when screened seats are available. The spectator has assumed the risks of being hit by a foul ball or released bat and cannot hold those in charge of the game liable.

Several concerns should be noted about this "defense." First, it is not a defense against negligence. The participant cannot release the person in charge of an activity from the duty of care owed to the participant, even if the form signed indicates such release. Public policy simply will not let persons who are responsible for the safety of those in their care shirk that duty to their participants. This defense is good only when there is no negligence. This defense applies when the plaintiff is claiming negligence but the injury actually resulted from a risk inherent in the activity of which the adult participant had full knowledge and voluntarily participated in the activity with that knowledge.

The second concern of this defense grows out of the first. Minors cannot except responsibility for protecting themselves from injury, and parents cannot waive their children's right to protection by persons in charge of activities in which their children are participating. Children are not seen as capable of recognizing the risks in activities. Likewise, people who are not mentally capable of recognizing the risks cannot be held responsible. Because minors and people with diminished mental capacity are unable to recognize risks, the onus is on those in charge of the activity to (1) remove or control existing risks to whatever extent possible, (2) warn participants of the remaining risks, and (3) instruct participants in ways to reduce or eliminate risks. This becomes part of the duty owed to participants. If these things are not present, the person in charge of the activity will be liable when injuries result from inherent risks of the activity.

Even adults who are capable of assuming the risks and of controlling their actions cannot be totally responsible for their injuries if there are hidden risks that are known to those offering the activity but of which the participant is not informed. People cannot assume a risk of which they are not aware. Again, the onus is on those in control to inform and instruct.

Exercise-related professionals should not take the above information as an indication that consent — express consent in particular — is of no value. An appropriately drafted participation agreement, for example, is one of the best ways to inform participants of the risks inherent in an activity. Agreements signed by a participant indicate that the participant

— understands and appreciates the risks involved in the activity;

— knows the safety rules and procedures, understands their importance, and agrees to comply with them; and

— is specifically requesting permission to participate in the activity.[2]

A properly drafted participation agreement cannot only show assumption of the risks; it also can be used to establish contributory or comparative negligence. If the participant violates something indicated in the agreement, the violation could be used to show lack of reasonableness and fault on the participant's part. (See Appendix A for a recommended format for a participation agreement.)

Act of God

3. *Act of God.* The "act of God" defense is based on the position that the injury was totally out of the control of anyone and therefore is attributable only to an act of God. As is the case with assumption of the risks, this defense is of little value in defending against negligence. It is of value only when negligence claims are brought in which there was no negligence. The defendant will claim that he did everything humanly possible to prevent accidents associated with the activity. He will claim that the accident that caused the injury was totally *unforeseeable*; therefore, he could have done nothing before or during the activity to prevent the injury.

People often think this defense is limited to occurrences in nature such as lightning bolts out of a blue sky. Although injuries that result from such occurrences certainly are within this category, the key here is foreseeability. Any accident that cannot be foreseen, and therefore cannot be planned for, will fall into this category. The mistake is to assume that accidents caused by occurrences in nature let those in charge of activities off the hook. Nothing could be farther from the truth. Lightning is a good example. When storm conditions are present, lightning is foreseeable and proper actions must be taken. If proper actions are not taken, the persons in charge of the activity are negligent and, therefore, liable for any resulting injury, even though lightning is "an act of God."

For the above "defenses" to be of any value to the professional who has been accused of negligence, the professional must not have been at fault at all or only partially at fault. The injured party bringing the claim must have contributed to her own injury, or the injury must have been the result of an inherent risk of the activity with no negligence on the professional's part, or something unforeseeable that could not have been controlled must have caused the injury. If the professional is at fault and that fault, even though unintentional, was the cause of an injury to a person in the care of the professional, the professional is liable for the injury to the participant and the losses incurred by the injured party as a result of the injury.

INTENTIONAL TORTS

Intentional tort

Unlike an unintentional tort, an intentional tort occurs as the result of some volition on the part of the tort-feasor. The tort-feasor either purposefully commits an act or purposefully fails to act, thereby resulting in some injury to an individual or an individual's property. U. S. society has decided that when one individual intentionally harms another, the person inflicting the harm should be punished. Intentional torts can be punished by bringing civil actions for damages or by bringing criminal charges that can result in a fine on the individual or by confining him to jail. Even though exercise-related professionals are less likely to commit intentional torts, some intentional torts should be mentioned as they are more likely to occur than others.

These intentional torts are battery, defamation, and false imprisonment. (A fourth intentional tort, intentional interference with a contractual right, will be discussed in Chapter 15.) Each of these torts has its own elements that must be proven against the alleged tort-feasor, but all must also include those elements that show intent. The general elements of intent are:

- a voluntary act or inaction,
- realization of the consequences of the act
- understanding that the consequences are the logical and likely results of the act.

Some might believe that intent is difficult to prove. One might ask, "How will anyone know whether I meant to do something or not?" Fortunately or unfortunately — depending which side of the case you are on — intent might not be that difficult to prove. There is no need to prove what was in a person's mind at the time of, or prior to the time of, the act that resulted in the injury. If an individual voluntarily does something or fails to do something and that action or lack of action has an obvious consequence that a reasonable person would expect, the elements of intent are almost a given. The perpetrator will have to prove that she could not have foreseen the consequences that any other reasonable person could have foreseen. With this in mind, the intentional torts listed above are discussed briefly in hopes that exercise-related professionals will be able to avoid acting in ways that could lead to claims of intentional torts against them.

Battery

Battery may be civil or criminal. The intent to harm is the difference. The elements of *civil battery* are

Battery

- Intent to contact
- Actual contact
- The contact is harmful or offensive
- The contact is unprivileged or unpermitted

The elements of *criminal battery* are

- Intent to harm through contact
- Actual contact
- The contact causes harm
- The contact was unprivileged or unpermitted

In the exercise-related professions, the contact the professionals have with the participants would rarely have the intent to harm. Therefore, the professionals would be unlikely to be charged with criminal battery. Civil battery is another story. There is certainly intent to contact, and contact occurs many times during the course of performing one's duties. Athletic trainers and therapists must touch their clients. Teachers and coaches are constantly touching their students and athletes to position them during drills and practices. Fitness and wellness specialists often touch participants to perform measurements and to assist them in performing exercises. In most cases, the main factors in determining civil battery are:

Was the contact harmful or offensive?

Was it done without privilege or permission?

In most cases, the contact of exercise-related professionals is performed with privilege. For example, the athletic trainer must touch the knee to wrap it. In this instance, the trainer has the privilege to contact the athlete to perform his duties. Such contact is not expected to cause any harm. In civil battery, however, harm is not necessary to prove battery. The contact only has to be offensive. If the trainer is constantly placing his hands on the inner thigh of the athlete when there is no need to do so or if the trainer places the athlete's foot in the trainer's crotch to wrap the knee, the athlete might find this offensive. The offensiveness might be magnified if the trainer and athlete are of the opposite sex.

If an athlete, or student, or client finds this type of touching offensive, it *is* offensive. If she brings a claim of civil battery, she need not prove that the offensiveness was intended. What must be shown is that there was intent to contact and that the resulting contact was offensive. A reasonable person should understand that a female athlete would be offended by having her foot placed in the crotch of a male trainer. The same can be said for the male or female coach patting players of the opposite sex on the buttocks after a good play or the teacher touching students inappropriately while spotting in gymnastics.

If exercise-related professionals are to avoid such charges, they must constantly be aware of the potential for their contact to be considered offensive. They should do only what is necessary to accomplish their tasks. If possible, females should work with females and males with males when the contact is likely to be in sensitive areas. If this is not possible, others should be present when such contact is necessary. As other tips:

- Establish habits and procedures that show concern and sensitivity for the feelings of others in such situations.

- Be professional in your dealings with participants when contact is necessary.

- Being friendly is one thing; joking inappropriately to the point of being crass is another. Be intelligent enough to know the difference.

None of this advice will guarantee against claims of battery, but it certainly will lower the possibility.

A special situation of potential battery deserves attention: Exercise-related professionals are responsible for the safety of their participants. This often involves protecting the participants from themselves and others. Crowds have to be controlled, fights may have to be broken up, one participant might threaten another or the professional might be threatened, or an outsider might threaten everyone. In these instances, forceful contact is likely — forceful enough to cause harm. The question is how *much* force can be used if necessary without being guilty of battery.

The rule of thumb is associated with self-defense. If the professional is the one being threatened because of another's action, he can defend himself by using reasonable force under the specific circumstances to repel the reasonably perceived threat of imminent violence. This means that if someone is attacking you with a baseball bat, you can use reasonable force to protect yourself and disarm the assailant as the circumstances dictate. You would not be expected to use the same force when the attacker is a second-grader as you would use when the attacker is a 250-pound adult. The same idea of reasonable force can be used in controlling an individual to prevent harm to others or to the individual being controlled.

Defamation

Defamation refers to spoken words (slander) and written words (libel) that are false and that hold the subject of the statement up to public ridicule. In addition to intent, the elements of defamation are (1) a false statement that is (2) published to a third party, (3) that holds the subject up to public ridicule, and thereby causes (4) financial loss. If the person being defamed is a public figure, a fifth element is added: (5) the act is done with malice or reckless disregard for the truth.

Defamation

People often say something about other people to third parties. It is done all the time in everyday conversation. This does not make it correct.

If something untrue is said about another that leads to that person losing her job or not getting a promotion, that person would have a claim of defamation against the publisher. To publish does not mean only to write. When we relay something to another either orally or in writing, we have published it. If you are in a management position and place something in a worker's file that is not true and that later plays a part in that worker's not getting a promotion, that worker has a claim of defamation against you. If you are asked to write a recommendation for a co-worker and make false statements in the recommendation that results in that person not getting the position applied for, that co-worker has a claim of defamation against you.

Public figure

If you make untrue statements about a public figure, that person would have to prove that you made the statements with malice or reckless disregard for the truth to have a claim of defamation against you. Who is a public figure? The easy answer is anyone elected to public office. Persons in public office must expect to be defamed about the job they are doing or are not doing. They must expect public ridicule. They have recourse against the defamer only when they can show that the defamer acted with total disregard for the truth. This can be easy when they can show that the defamer had "actual notice" of the truth and chose to publish the false information instead. Otherwise, the public official will have a difficult time proving defamation.

Persons other than public officials also can be public figures, but it is not always easy to identify them as such. If, because of their occupation, the person has assumed a certain position in society or taken a certain stance on issues, that person might be considered a public official. Well-known college coaches who make it a point to be in the news and in the public eye regularly might be considered public figures, although all coaches are certainly not public figures. Well-known physicians who choose to advertise their practices or voice their opinions about important health issues might be public figures, although not all physicians are public figures.

Of course, there is really no concern about who is a public official and who is not if you simply refrain from telling untruths about anyone. The truth is an absolute defense against defamation. You can publish anything about anyone no matter how vile, as long as it is the truth. You might also have a qualified privilege to say what you have said. A *qualified privilege* exists when the statement is made with no reason to believe it was false and is made by someone with a reason to make it to someone with a justifiable interest in knowing.

The most common example of this is when a witness gives information to a policeman that turns out to be false. If the witness was giving information she thought was true, the person against whom the information was about has no claim of defamation. If the opposite were the case, no witnesses would ever come forward, for fear of being sued for defamation if by chance they were incorrect.

An example more closely related to the professional is an example used earlier. Managers often have the responsibility of passing on information to others in the form of recommendations. They might include information in the recommendation that they have every reason to believe is true but the information turns out to be false. Because the information was provided only to someone who had a justifiable reason to know this information, the manager would not be guilty of defamation as long as he could show that he had no way of knowing the information was false.

False Imprisonment

The elements of false imprisonment are when individuals are (1) intentionally detained or confined (2) without their consent (3) by someone without privilege or permission (4) for an appreciable length of time, thereby denying them the right to go where they want to go. Will an exercise-related professional ever have the privilege to confine another? If you are a coach and two of your athletes get in an argument in which one threatens the other, would you have the privilege to confine to your office the athlete who made the threat while she cooled down even though she resisted being placed there? The answer is a qualified "yes." You have that privilege as long as you do not use excessive force to place her there and as long as you do not keep her there too long. Your privilege arises from the duty of your position to protect your players from harm and to use reasonable means to do so.

False imprisonment

What if you manage a fitness club and you see a member leaving with a bag of equipment that belongs to the club? Can you detain him until you determine whether he is stealing the equipment? The answer depends on the jurisdiction in which you are located. In some jurisdictions, your only recourse is to call the police and report a theft. In others, you might be able to make use of the *shopkeeper's privilege*. This is a law that has been passed in some jurisdictions giving the business owner the privilege to detain a customer if the shopkeeper (1) has a reasonable suspicion that the customer is stealing something, (2) provided that the detention is for a reasonable period of time, (3) the shopkeeper uses only reasonable force to detain the customer, and (4) the customer is retrieved only from a reasonable distance.

Shopkeeper's privilege

Would the manager be guilty of false imprisonment for detaining the club member in the above example? First, if the club member were really stealing the equipment, the manager would not be guilty of false imprisonment. If someone else had lent the equipment to the member without telling the manager, however, the manager's guilt would depend on how she handled the situation. If she simply stopped the member while he was still in the club and detained him long enough to verify his story about someone lending him the equipment, there would be no false imprisonment. If, however, she ran down the member in the parking lot, dragged him back into the club, and physically held him down while she had someone call the police and then waited for the police to arrive only to find that someone had lent the member the equipment, she would probably be guilty of false imprisonment.

To avoid being accused of false imprisonment, you should not overreact, do what you would expect a reasonable person to do in such cases, and do only what would be expected of your position. The shopkeeper should keep one other thing in mind. If he treats the person he suspects of stealing in a way that publishes to others that this individual is a thief and it turns out that she is not, the suspected thief might sue the shopkeeper for defamation as well as false imprisonment. This is another good reason not to overreact.

RECAP

If you commit a wrong against another resulting in injury to that person or that person's property, you are guilty of a tort. That tort may be criminal, or it may be civil in nature. If it is criminal, the State will bring you to trial and impose a fine against you or put you in jail if you are found guilty. If it is a civil tort, the injured party, the plaintiff, will sue you, the defendant, for damages.

Even though exercise-related professionals might find themselves facing criminal charges, they are more likely to face a civil suit for failing to meet their duty to their clients, students, or athletes. Because doctrines such as sovereign immunity no longer protect the state and legal defenses such as contributory negligence no longer totally exonerate the tort-feasor, more and more suits are being brought against persons who fail to meet their standard of care. In the United States, our concept of fault demands that the tort-feasor make the injured party whole again. This applies to those directly responsible and to those indirectly, or vicariously, responsible. Those found responsible are liable for actual damages and may also be liable for speculative and punitive damages.

Torts also may be intentional or unintentional. Unintentional torts are torts of negligence — failure of parties to do what reasonable persons in their position should have done either through commission or omission. For injured parties to prove negligence against another, they must establish that there was a duty owed, that duty was breached, and the breach was the proximate cause of an actual injury for which the suit is being brought. If injured parties can also show that the tort-feasor acted with wanton or intentional disregard for the injured parties' safety, they can show gross negligence and seek punitive damages, provided there were actual damages.

When faced with a negligence claim, alleged tort-feasors' best defense is to prove there was no negligence by showing that they did their duty and if there was an injury, it did not result from any breach of that duty. Short of that, alleged tort-feasors might attempt to show that the injured party contributed to his own injury, totally or in part. They might also show that the injury was one that might be expected and that the injured party had assumed the risk of such injuries. Alleged tort-feasors could also show that the injury was an act of God that was totally unforeseeable. In either case, negligence would not exist.

Intentional torts are voluntary acts of the tort-feasor that are offensive or result in harm to another. The more common intentional torts that exercise-related professionals face are battery, defamation, false imprisonment, and intentional interference with a contractual right. In each of these torts, the elements of intent, as well as elements specific to the tort, must be proven. Proving intent can be as simple as showing that tort-feasors should have known, as reasonable persons, that their actions would cause what they did cause. And because their actions were voluntary, there was intent to cause what was obvious. The best way to avoid intentional torts is to think rationally and act reasonably. If you fail to do either of these, you may find yourself charged with an intentional tort or an unintentional tort.

NOTES

1. N. J. Dougherty et al. (1994). *Sport, Physical Activity, and the Law.* Champaign, IL: Human Kinetics.

2. Dougherty.

RESOURCES

Appenzeller, H. (Ed.) (1985). *Sports and Law, Contemporary Issues.* Charlottesville, VA: Michie Co.

Carpenter, L. J. (1995). *Legal Concepts in Sport: A Primer.* Reston, VA: American Alliance for Health, Physical Education, Recreation and Dance.

Nolan, J. R., and J. M. Nolan-Haley (1990). *Black's Law Dictionary*, 6th ed. St. Paul: West Publishing.

Constitutional Law

OBJECTIVES

After studying this chapter, you should be able to:

1. Identify individual rights guaranteed by the U.S. Constitution and give an example of how each one might be violated in the exercise-related professions.

2. Discuss the importance of the Fourteenth Amendment in extending individual rights.

3. Define state actors and give examples of state actors.

4. Discuss under what conditions state actors might legally violate individual constitutional rights.

5. Define and give examples of fundamental rights.

6. Identify specific groups the courts have recognized as "suspect classifications."

7. Identify conditions under which a state actor might require a drug test for participants and/or employees.

8. Identify at least five federal laws that extend constitutional protections to segments of society other than state actors, and give examples of how these affect the exercise-related professions.

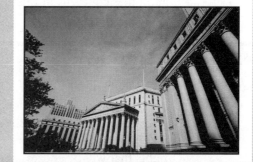

Constitutional rights and laws associated with those rights cover a wide variety of issues. We cannot cover all of these issues here. Only those that are most closely associated with the exercise-related professions will be addressed. Many of the issues associated with our constitutional rights are points of concern in the exercise-related professions today. Equal opportunity for everyone to participate in sports and in employment in all venues regardless of gender, race, age, or disability, and equal pay for equal work regardless of gender, are issues as relevant today as they were prior to the 1960s. The requirements for drug testing, in athletic participation and in employment in general, stretch to their limits our rights to freedom from unwarranted searches and seizures and the right not to testify against ourselves. The right not to be sexually harassed in the workplace, at school, or on athletic teams is constantly in today's headlines. And the right to due process before being released from our jobs has never been more critical than today, when downsizing is seen as the key to survival and buy-outs and relocations are a way of life in the business world. We will examine these and other concerns in this chapter.

CONSTITUTIONAL RIGHTS

Constitutional rights

Individual constitutional rights are granted to us in the first 10 amendments to the U.S. Constitution. Known as the Bill of Rights, these 10 amendments were added to the Constitution in 1791 and provide that the U.S. Congress will pass no laws that abridge the rights delineated therein. The individual rights that will be addressed in this text are:

— the right to free exercise of religion and the right to freedom of speech (First Amendment)

— the right to be free from unwarranted searches and seizures (Fourth Amendment)

— the right not to testify against oneself (Fifth Amendment)

— the right not to be deprived of life, liberty, or property without due process of law (Fifth and Fourteenth Amendments)

— the right to equal protection under the law (Fourteenth Amendment). (See Appendix B.)

From 1791 until 1868, the Bill of Rights protected U.S. citizens only from laws made by the U.S. Congress. Individual states could pass laws that abridged individual rights in any way they wished as long as this was not prohibited by the states' constitutions and did not deal with an area of law reserved for the federal government. This was changed in 1868, when the Fourteenth Amendment was added to the U.S. Constitution. This amendment passed along to state governments the prohibition against enacting or enforcing any laws that abridged individual rights granted to U.S. citizens. It included a specific statement preventing the states from depriving a citizen of life, liberty, or property without due process of law. In addition to those two statements, another important right was added: No state can deny to any person within its jurisdiction equal protection of the laws.

The Fourteenth Amendment has no wording that extends these prohibitions to governmental entities other than the states. Over time, however, the courts, through precedent-setting cases, have determined that all levels of government (municipal, county, district, borough, and so on) are extensions of the State and, therefore, are subject to the prohibitions of the first 10 amendments through the Fourteenth Amendment. In some cases, the prohibitions have been extended to any entity that acts in a governmental manner. For example, the National Collegiate Athletic Association is an apparently private entity that has been held to the prohibitions in some situations.

These prohibitions also have been extended to cover regulations and rules of governmental entities. As mentioned in Chapter 12, regulations are often formulated to enforce laws. Because of this, the regulation carries the force of law. This can result in the regulation's restricting individual rights, so the courts have decided that the regulations must also be subject to the prohibitions. Likewise, rules that governmental entities put into place to govern conduct might limit access to their services or abridge individual rights. This is especially true in governmental entities such as public schools, state colleges and universities, and public recreational programs.

ABRIDGING CONSTITUTIONAL RIGHTS

None of the amendments contains language indicating that the governmental entities can abridge individual rights under certain circumstances. The courts, however, (again through their precedent-setting decisions), have established a complex system under which governmental entities can enact and enforce laws that do violate the prohibitions of the first 10 and the Fourteenth Amendments. Having a basic understanding of this system is important, first, because we are all subject to laws passed by these bodies as citizens and, second, because we might be charged with implementing these laws as public employees.

Before looking at the system for determining when governmental entities can abridge our rights, we reiterate that we are talking about governmental or *state actors* only. State actors are the federal government, state government, and any subunit of these two governments. Only these entities have promised not to abridge our rights through the Constitution. Private businesses and corporations have made no such promise and are generally free to violate individual rights unless they are subject to specific laws that have been enacted to prevent such violation. These laws will be discussed later in this chapter.

State actors

State actors can violate our individual rights if the laws they pass are rationally related to a legitimate State interest unless the right being violated by the law is a *fundamental right*. If the right being violated is a fundamental right, the law must be necessary to accomplish a compelling State interest. Rationally related? Legitimate State interest? Fundamental right? Compelling State interest? What is all of this gobbledygook, and who determines what each of these terms means? *Who* determines is the easy answer. The courts determine whether a law is violating our rights without being rationally related to a legitimate State interest or without being necessary to accomplish a compelling State interest.

Fortunately or unfortunately, this typically happens only after laws and regulations have been enacted and have been allowed to violate our rights. An individual (or group of individuals) eventually decides that the law is violating some right and takes the state actor to court for having an unconstitutional law. As an example, suppose a state decides that the number of athletic trainers in the state is increasing too rapidly and this increase is accompanied by a decline in the quality of the service the trainers provide. In an attempt to control the number of athletic trainers, the state passes a law requiring all new trainers to weigh at least 225 pounds. The state actor rationalizes that too many of the trainers are having difficulty moving and working with athletes who appear to be getting larger and larger every year. Athletic trainers already working in the state are "grandfathered" in so none lose their job. Other than the obvious facetiousness of such a law, what are the problems?

If someone believes this law is having a *disparate impact* on her and, therefore, that the law is unconstitutional, she can take the State to court. The person who believes her rights are being violated challenges the constitutionality of the law in court, and the State presents its reasoning as to why the law meets a legitimate or compelling State interest. The court decides the constitutionality of the law by determining whether the State has succeeded in justifying the law.

Fundamental Rights

The first question to be answered is whether a fundamental right is involved. If it is, the State's rationale must meet a higher standard. In essence, the State must clear a higher hurdle. If a fundamental right is not involved, the law needs only to be rationally related to a legitimate State interest — a lower hurdle.

Fundamental rights

What are our fundamental rights? Black's *Legal Dictionary* defines fundamental rights as "those rights which have their source, and are explicitly or implicitly guaranteed, in the federal constitution . . . and state constitutions." Rights explicitly guaranteed in the Constitution are fairly easy to determine. We read them there as the right to freedom of speech, free exercise of religion, the right to bear arms, freedom from unwarranted searches and seizures, and so on. Even though some still argue about exactly what these rights mean, most of us have a definite feeling as to what they mean to each of us individually. Some of the other explicit rights are not so clear.

What exactly does the right not to "be deprived of life, liberty, or property without due process of law" mean? It is fairly obvious that it means a state actor cannot take your life without going through the appropriate procedures of law from the time you are arrested and charged through whatever appeals processes are available to you. It also means that the law you have been charged with violating and the procedures followed when you are charged must be fair. That is a well-established fundamental right.

Due process of law

It also means that a state actor cannot deprive you of your property rights without following an appropriate and fair process. The courts have interpreted property rights to include more than a piece of dirt or any other tangible item you might own. You have property rights in intangible things as well — such as the expectancies you have related to your employment. If a state actor has hired you to work for a year, you have an expectancy to work for a full year. You have a property right in the salary and benefits you expect over that period. The state actor cannot arbitrarily take this right away from you without due process. Could this be a possible problem with the state law example given above? Do those prospective athletic trainers who cannot get a job in this particular state because they weigh less than 225 pounds have a property right in a job for which they are yet to be hired? Are those already on the job in jeopardy of losing their jobs because of the law?

Another explicitly guaranteed right that is not so easily understood is the right that prevents a state from denying any person in its jurisdiction equal protection of the law. When we think of this right, we typically think of being treated equally by law enforcement personnel. We do not expect police officers to treat one individual or a group of individuals different from any other individual or group. Although this is certainly part of this right, the right goes much further. Even though this is an explicit guarantee, this right is the source of many of our implicit rights as determined by the courts. Any law that would cause one person or a group of persons to be treated different from others would be in violation of this right.

Equal protection of the law

Laws that would impede the right of one group to travel freely between states or laws that would allow one person or group to be discriminated against when being considered for a job would be laws creating unequal protection and, therefore, would violate this fundamental right. This right is responsible for preventing discrimination by state actors. Does this right create a problem for the State in the athletic trainer's law above? Is the State discriminating against persons who are qualified athletic trainers but cannot get a job in this state because they weigh less than 225 pounds? Maybe so, or maybe not, because this brings into question another layer of the system the courts set up for determining whether states are within their rights in enacting certain laws.

"Suspect" Classification

Suspect classification

This right of equal protection has traditionally not been as inviolable as other rights, as states must pass laws all the time that would seem to be discriminatory to certain groups. States must still have a rational reason for enacting such laws, but they do not have to go beyond a rational reason unless certain circumstances are present. This requires asking a second question: Is the individual or group of individuals affected by the law a protected or "suspect" classification? The courts have decided that when laws seem to have an effect on certain groups, those laws are immediately suspect as discriminatory because this group has been discriminated against so much in the past.

The courts have identified several suspect classifications, including race, alienage, and national origin. Laws that have a disparate impact on any of these three classifications are permitted only if the law is necessary to accomplish a compelling State interest. This now requires the State to jump the same hurdle that it must clear when a law affects a fundamental right. In the example of the athletic trainer, qualified athletic trainers weighing less than 225 pounds would seem to be the group being discriminated against. They do not qualify as a suspect class.

The courts recently placed two other classifications in an elevated status regarding equal protection of the law. These two classifications — gender and disability — have not attained suspect classification status. The courts have said that states enacting laws that have a disparate impact on a gender or on persons who have disabilities must have something more than a rational reason for a legitimate State interest for enacting the law. This "something more" does not have to reach the level of being necessary to accomplish a compelling State interest. The reasoning is somewhere in between these two hurdles: Exactly *where* will be determined by the courts case by case. Does the athletic trainer law have a problem here? A problem is not immediately obvious from the wording of the law *per se*, but will this law have a disparate impact on women?

Let's say it does, because fewer qualified female athletic trainers will reach the 225-pound cut-off than will qualified male athletic trainers. If qualified female trainers who weigh less than 225 pounds apply for the jobs and do not get them, they might sue the State individually or as a class. They will at least claim violation of their right to equal protection of the law, and the law must be something more than rationally related to a legitimate State interest. Now comes the next step in the analysis as to whether the law is constitutional or not.

Legitimate and Compelling Interest

Does the state have at least a legitimate interest that it is protecting, and does its interest rise to the compelling level if necessary? The State has an interest in ensuring that its citizens get the best athletic training care possible. If there had been no interest, the legislators would not have enacted this law in the first place. Is the interest legitimate? States certainly have a responsibility to protect their citizens. This state may even be one that requires athletic trainers to be licensed and not just certified. The State requires licensure because it wants more control over athletic training practitioners by setting rules and standards for being licensed to be employed and for having the license revoked and employment terminated when the rules and standards are not met.

Safety and care of the state's athletes, especially those who are minors in public school athletic programs, are definitely a legitimate State interest. Because the State has taken the responsibility to ensure quality care for its citizens who are athletes, the State could be sued for licensing substandard athletic trainers to practice in the state. This could easily elevate their interest to the compelling level. This law probably meets and exceeds the tests of legitimate State interest. But there is one more hurdle to cross.

Rational Relationship

The state now must answer the question: Is the law rationally related to the State's legitimate interest? The State must show that weighing less than 225 pounds prevents an athletic trainer from providing quality care to athletes. It also must show that weighing 225 pounds or more will improve the quality of care to athletes. If the State can do this to the satisfaction of the court, it might win. The females who brought the suit will also be presenting evidence that counters the evidence the State presents. The court will weigh the two arguments and decide who wins.

This procedure will be followed in any situation where individuals challenge a law or other action by a state actor that they believe is unconstitutional because it violates their rights. Future exercise-related professionals might find themselves in positions to either have their rights violated as employees or to violate the rights of others as program providers. Many exercise-related positions are available in the public sector. Therefore, many of the persons preparing in this field will eventually work for State entities. Examples of these positions are exercise scientists, physical education teachers, recreators, coaches, sport managers, athletic trainers, and wellness personnel in state colleges and universities; physical education teachers, coaches, athletic trainers, and athletic directors in public schools; recreators, managers, fitness specialists, and coaches in public recreation departments and fitness centers; and athletic trainers, therapists, and wellness/fitness specialists in state and federally run hospitals and clinics. As the rights below are presented, consider how a state actor might violate your individual rights or how you might violate another's rights if you are employed by a state actor.

FIRST AMENDMENT RIGHTS

First Amendment rights include the free exercise of religion and freedom of speech and expression.

Free Exercise of Religion

In the area of freedom of religion, state entities cannot formulate policies that (1) endorse or advance a religious belief or practice, (2) place a burden on the free exercise of another's religion by forcing him to choose between his religious requirements and requirements he must meet in their programs, or (3) have the effect of treating an individual (or group) unequally simply because of her religion.

State entities such as public schools are most likely to violate these rights. Requirements in physical education classes, such as wearing specific types of clothing or participating in activities that entail close contact between males and females might violate a student's rights. Practices such as prayers before games or during assemblies might also be a violation.

Hiring practices might come into question for any state entity if religious practices seem to be used in selecting employees for certain positions. (It should be noted here that the courts have also considered religion as a "suspect class.") Can you think of specific examples where public entities might violate one or more of these conditions?

Freedom of Speech/Expression

Even though the Constitution guarantees U.S. citizens freedom of speech, the courts have determined that this speech can be reasonably restricted as to time, place, and manner, as long as such restrictions do not eliminate freedom of speech or expression altogether. Physical education teachers, athletic trainers, and coaches at the public grade-school level and in public colleges and universities should be particularly aware of their students' and athletes' right to freedom of expression. Public recreators should also be aware that they could violate this right by establishing restrictive policies or rules concerning behavior of participants.

Is this to say that no rules can be established concerning what students, athletes, and recreation participants can wear or say while in school, on an athletic team, or participating in recreational programs? Certainly not. State courts have consistently upheld school and municipal policies that prevent students/participants from wearing clothing with statements or pictures that are profane or lewd or degrading to others. The U. S. Supreme Court has not overturned these state court decisions.

If you are in the position to impose restrictive policies or rules that might abridge one's freedom of speech or expression, you can restrict the type of speech that would cause disruptions or could be considered socially inappropriate (especially in public schools, which have the responsibility to teach the boundaries of socially appropriate behavior). Nevertheless, you cannot restrict speech or expression simply because it is unpopular or controversial. Can you give examples in which public entities are allowed to restrict freedom of speech or expression and examples of restrictions that might be in violation of this right?

FOURTH AMENDMENT RIGHTS

The right of freedom from unwarranted search and seizure is related to one's expectancy of privacy for his person, in his possessions, and in his home. It is most often thought of in relation to the police's need to have a valid search warrant to search our homes for evidence related to a crime. Because exercise-related professionals will have no need to search an individual's home, they are most likely to encounter this right in relation to the individual's person and possessions.

Exercise-related professionals as officials working for public entities might have reason to search an individual's person for drugs or weapons. They also might have reason to search an individual's possessions (a book bag, a purse, a sport bag, or a locker) for this material. Can they do this without a valid search warrant? In the case of school officials, the answer is "yes." The school official must have a *reasonable suspicion* that the search will reveal evidence that the student has violated a school rule (or the law). The search must be both *reasonable in its inception* and *reasonable in its scope*. These guidelines apply to searching the person of the individual, anything she is carrying, such as a book bag, and to her locker (as long as the locker is considered the property of the institution and not the property of the individual).

Whether public officials such as recreational managers would or would not have this same "privilege" has not been determined. Because they have the same responsibility for the safety of their participants and often have the same type of rules concerning possession of weapons and use of drugs, it is difficult to believe they could not use the same methods to safeguard their participants and programs.

Exercise-related professionals might also require a drug test for employment or participation. Drug tests are considered a search of one's person. The courts have upheld drug tests required by public entities for employment when the use of drugs would present a safety hazard (for example, drugs would impair the functioning of someone hired as a public transportation driver and present a safety hazard to passengers and others).

The courts also have upheld drug tests required for participation in athletics (in public schools, colleges and universities, and other public amateur athletic venues). In this area the test must have met one of the following stipulations:

1. The test was given with the athlete's written consent.
2. The test must have been reasonable (focused on specific persons with supportive facts).
3. The test was conducted subject to a valid search warrant.

Most drug-testing programs for athletic participation depend on obtaining the athlete's consent to the testing. Of course, this means "no consent, no play." Even though the courts have said that coercion cannot be used to obtain consent, they have also said that "no consent, no play" is not coercive, even when it means losing a scholarship. Can you think of ways in which an exercise-related professional might violate an individual's right to freedom from an unwarranted search or seizure?

FIFTH AMENDMENT RIGHTS

Fifth Amendment rights incorporate the right not to be witness against the self and the right not to be deprived of life, liberty, and the pursuit of happiness.

The Right Not to be a Witness Against Oneself

The right not to be a witness against the self in the exercise-related professions comes into play in conjunction with the Fourth Amendment right mentioned above. Results of a drug test would be considered testifying against oneself and could not be used in a criminal trial against an individual (unless obtained by a valid warrant). Most, if not all, cases of drug testing for athletic participation will involve no warrant in the drug-testing procedure. Because the purpose for drug testing in these situations is to determine whether an individual is abiding by the rules of the organization, criminal charges are generally not a consideration. The information provided to prospective participants concerning drug testing should state exactly how the results of the test will be used and that such use will be restricted to declaring the participant ineligible. This will avoid problems with the individual's Fifth Amendment rights.

The Right Not to be Deprived of Life, Liberty, or Property without Due Process of Law

As mentioned above, *due process* refers to both the reason we might be deprived of our life, liberty, or property and to the procedure through which we are deprived. When we are accused of violating these rules and laws, we expect our rules and laws to be fair and we expect to be treated fairly. In the exercise-related professions, we are most likely to be involved in due process questions in relation to loss of property rights. The expectancies of a job or the expectancies of a scholarship are considered property rights.

To ensure that rules are fair, administrators of exercise-related programs should formulate only rules that (1) have a valid purpose or function, (2) are applied in such a way that the application is clearly related to accomplishing the purpose, and (3) are clear and concise with no ambiguity. To ensure that the procedures followed are fair if someone is accused of violating a rule or is otherwise in jeopardy of losing a property right (such as being fired), the guideline for administrators is:[1] Where the severity of the violation and the severity of the sanction to be imposed are low, *minimum* due process should include:

Minimum due process

1. A statement of the specific violation.
2. Some notice of what sanctions will be imposed.
3. An opportunity for the accused to comment on the action.

As the severity of the violation and the sanction to be imposed increases, guarding the rights of the affected individual becomes more important and requires a more specific procedure to be followed. In these cases, *maximum* due process procedures would be:[2]

Maximum due process

1. Written notice of an impartial hearing where charges and facts will be presented.
2. A written statement of the charges and the grounds that, if proven, would justify the imposition of sanctions.
3. Provision of an adversarial hearing (which would include the assistance of legal counsel in the more serious cases).

4. A written or taped record of the proceedings of the hearing.

5. A clearly stated right of appeal if the results are adverse to the person affected.

FOURTEENTH AMENDMENT RIGHTS

The Fourteenth Amendment promises U. S. citizens the right to equal protection of the law, meaning that all persons will be treated equally under the laws of each state. This promise is what protects us from discrimination based on who we are. As mentioned, the courts have identified race, alienage, and national origin, as well as religion, as suspect classes. Therefore, any disparate treatment with a basis in one of these classes must be necessary to accomplish a compelling State interest. Although not identified as suspect classes, the court has recognized gender and disability as classifications requiring potentially discriminating legislation to need something more than simply being rationally related to a legitimate State interest.

Administrators in the exercise-related professions must assure that their rules and practices do not discriminate against these classes of individuals. If discrimination does exist, it must be based on a compelling State interest. Rules and practices related to participation, access to services, hiring and firing, retention, promotion, and demotion are likely areas for discrimination to appear in all professions. If these professions are in public entities, persons affected can bring action under the Fourteenth Amendment, or they can bring action under one of numerous laws passed to prevent discrimination. An important aspect of these laws is that they extend the constitutional protection of equal treatment under the law beyond public entities. Under certain conditions, private entities are also subject to these laws.

LAWS THAT EXTEND CONSTITUTIONAL PROTECTIONS BEYOND STATE ACTORS

The following is a discussion of laws that the federal government has passed to combat discrimination. (Most states have passed similar laws.) We cannot discuss in detail the origin and impact of each of these laws. Suffice it to say that these laws have had a significant impact on the exercise-related professions and will continue to do so.

Civil Rights Act of 1964

The Civil Rights Act of 1964 prevents discrimination based on race, color, or national origin in access to places of public accommodation (Title II) and in access to services and programs that are federally funded (Title VI). This act also prevents discrimination on the basis of race, color, national origin, gender, and religion in employment practices of employers that employ 15 or more people (Title VII).

Title II

Title II of the Civil Rights Act reaches virtually all aspects of U.S. society. The only organizations that are not public accommodations are private clubs that meet specific standards. The first standard that must be met is that the organization cannot be involved in interstate commerce. This is a difficult standard to meet and, therefore, few organizations are true private clubs.

Title VI

Most agencies and organizations subject to Title VI of the Civil Rights Act are public agencies that receive federal funds. These agencies are already expected to be nondiscriminatory under the Fourteenth Amendment. Some agencies that provide exercise-related programs might also receive federal funds through special grants or through federal contracts.

Title VII

Title VII has become a major weapon in employment discrimination, not only in the exercise-related occupations but in all occupations. All employers with 15 or more employees are subject to this law. Even though it has been used extensively to provide equal opportunity for all persons in employment, Title VII is probably best known today for its association with *sexual harassment* claims. The Civil Rights Act says there shall be no discrimination in the "conditions" of employment for any individual. "Conditions" have been interpreted to mean virtually any aspect of employment. Therefore, employers are restricted from making sexual favors a condition of continuing employment, raises, promotion, and the like. Employers are also responsible for ensuring that the "sexual environment" is not of a condition such that it would negatively affect the performance of any employee.

Educational Amendments Act of 1972

Title IX of the Educational Amendments provides that no person shall, on the basis of sex, be excluded from participation in, be denied the benefits of, or be subjected to discrimination under any education program or activity receiving federal funds. This law impacts on all educational programs, both public and private, at all levels that receive federal funds. If only one program of many at a school receives federal funds, all programs at the school, not just the program receiving the funds, must adhere to this law.

This law significantly affects physical education, athletic training, and sports programs at all levels of education. This is the law responsible for coeducational physical education and the growth of sport programs for girls at the grade school and college/university levels. Title IX requires programs for males and females to be commensurate in each of the following areas:

athletic financial assistance	practice and competitive facilities
accommodation of interests and abilities	medical and training facilities and services
equipment and supplies	housing
scheduling of games and practice times	dining facilities and services
travel and per-diem allowance	publicity
tutors	support services
coaches	recruitment of student athletes
locker rooms	

Some of these areas apply to athletics at the college/university level only.

Athletes are not employees. Therefore, they cannot bring charges of sexual harassment against coaches, athletic directors, and institutions under the sections of the Civil Rights Act mentioned above. Because Title IX is a nondiscrimination law, though, and because sexual harassment is a form of gender discrimination, athletes who are subjected to sexual harassment as an athlete can bring such charges under Title IX.

What athletic programs must do to be in compliance with Title IX are not found in the law itself. The requirements are found in the Policy Interpretations to the law. If the exercise-related profession you have chosen is coaching or athletic administration, you should make sure you are familiar with these requirements.

Rehabilitation Act of 1973

Section 504 of the Rehabilitation Act of 1973 states that no qualified handicapped person shall, on the basis of handicap, be excluded from participation in, be denied the benefits of, or otherwise be subjected to discrimination under any program or activity that receives or benefits from federal financial assistance. This law prevents discrimination for all persons with disabilities in employment, education, health, social services, or any other program, including recreational and sports programs, that receive *or benefit from* federal funds. The person with disabilities must be qualified for the job or be eligible to participate in the services or programs in question. "Qualified" assumes that some reasonable accommodation might have to be made for the person to do a specific job or to participate in a specific program.

In the case of recreation and sports programs at local levels, the "benefit from" language of this law is important. Many local recreation and sports programs might not receive federal funds today, but they play on fields or courts that exist only because of federal money that was made available to improve recreational facilities in that locale.

Americans with Disabilities Act of 1990

The Americans with Disabilities Act (ADA) prohibits discrimination in public accommodations for all persons with disabilities. This law, using the "public accommodation" language of the Civil Rights Act of 1964, extends the prohibitions of the Rehabilitation Act of 1973 to entities other than those receiving or benefiting from federal funds. As mentioned above, public accommodations are entities that do not meet the criteria for designation as a private club. This law affects exercise-related professionals in a wide variety of areas such as health services, health spas, places of exercise, gymnasiums, and most health and fitness facilities.

Individuals with Disabilities Education Act of 1990

The Individuals with Disabilities Education Act (IDEA) provides for free education of children with disabilities in the least restrictive environment without discrimination based on their disability. Even though the Rehabilitation Act of 1973 guaranteed access to educational programs for people with disabilities, it was thought that that law did not go far enough. The 1990 law requires *individualized education programs* (IEPs) complete with supplemental aids and related services where necessary.

The service related to physical education for students with disabilities is usually physical therapy. If children cannot participate in a physical education class at some level, they can still benefit from physical movement through physical therapy. School physical education and extracurricular programs are specifically defined in this law as areas where integration will be made in the least restrictive environment, with progressive placement in less restrictive environments as necessary.

Equal Pay Act of 1973 and 1982

The Equal Pay Acts provide that there shall be no discrimination on the basis of gender by paying lower wages to employees of one sex for work requiring equal skill, effort, and responsibility and performed under similar working conditions at the same place. This law applies to all private and public employers subject to the Fair Labor Standards Act (which are all employers covered by minimum wage and overtime laws). This law is of special interest to female coaches who get paid less than their male counterparts when they have equal experience and equivalent job requirements.

Equal Employment Opportunity Act of 1972

The Equal Employment Opportunity Act is an amendment to the Civil Rights Act of 1964. This law prevents discrimination in hiring practices based on race, color, gender, religion, or national origin, except where religion, gender, or national origin is a bona fide occupational qualification and is reasonably necessary to the conduct of a particular business. This law applies to all employers of 15 or more employees for each working day in each of 20 or more calendar weeks in a current or preceding calendar year.

As can be seen from this brief review of laws, the equal treatment promised to U.S. citizens from federal entities has been extended to many private entities. In addition to extending equal treatment, due process concerns are extended to private entities through contract law. Contract law will be discussed in Chapter 15.

NOTES

1. N. J. Dougherty, et al. *Sport, Physical Activity, and the Law* (Champaign, IL: Human Kinetics Publishers, 1994).

2. Dougherty, et al.

RESOURCES

Americans with Disabilities Act of 1990. 42 U.S.C. 12101.

Appenzeller, H. (Ed.) (1985). *Sports and Law: Contemporary Issues.* Charlottesville, VA: Michie Co.

Bethel School District No. 403 v. Fraser. 478 U.S. 675 (1986).

Carpenter, L. J. (1995). *Legal Concepts in Sport: A Primer.* Reston, VA: American Alliance for Health, Physical Education, Recreation and Dance.

Civil Rights Act of 1964. 42 U.S.C. 1985.

Educational Amendment Act of 1972 (PL 92–318, 86 Stat. 373). 20 U.S.C. 1681.

Equal Pay Act. 29 U.S.C. 206.

Individuals with Disabilities Act. 20 U.S.C. 1406 (1982).

Individuals with Disabilities Education Act. 20 U.S.C. 1232.

New Jersey v. T. L. O., 469 U. S. 325, 105 S. CT. 733 (1985).

Nolan, J. R., and J. M. Nolan-Haley, (1990). *Black's Law Dictionary*, 6th ed. St. Paul: West Publishing.

Rehabilitation Act of 1973. 29 U.S.C. 701.

Tinker v. Des Moines Independent School District. 393 U.S. 503 (1969).

Vernonia School District 47J v. Acton. 515 U. S. 646 (1995).

Contract Law

OBJECTIVES

After studying this chapter, you should be able to:

1. List and discuss the six elements of an enforceable contract.

2. Recognize the difference between a counteroffer and an acceptance when bargaining.

3. Describe the difference between a void and a voidable contract.

4. Give at least one example each of a breach of contract for a sale of goods and an employment contract.

5. Discuss "specific performance" and damages as remedies to a breach of contract.

6. Define *caveat emptor* and *caveat vendor* and discuss the significance of the difference between the two.

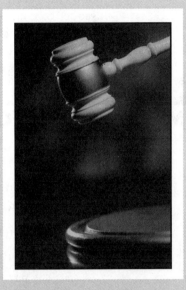

7. Identify the two implied warranties provided by the Uniform Commercial Code and discuss their importance to the purchaser of goods.

8. Identify the differences between being hired as an independent contractor and a full-time employee.

9. Identify the three typical reasons that employers use to show cause for terminating personnel contracts.

Administrators in the exercise-related professions typically deal with contracts in two areas: contracting for personal services and contracting for the purchase of goods. In both situations, the act of contracting is *an agreement between two or more persons that creates an obligation to do or not to do a given thing*. The key words in this statement are "agreement" and "obligation." The two parties of the contract agree to obligate themselves to one another. Once the agreement has been made, the parties go about meeting the responsibilities to which they have obligated themselves.

As long as everyone is happy with what the other parties to the contract are doing, there is generally little problem. If a test-grade treadmill has been ordered and one built for regular activity use is delivered, however, the receiving party believes the sender has not lived up to his obligations and a disagreement might arise between the two parties. The receiving party thinks he is being shorted on the equipment and will demand the sending party to meet her obligations. If the sending party claims no error has been made and makes no effort to rectify the situation, the receiving party will usually seek a legal remedy by taking the sender to court. The court will first interpret the agreement between the two parties to determine whether an agreement does or does not exist. If an agreement does exist, the court will then determine who has and who has not met his or her obligations.

ELEMENTS OF AN ENFORCEABLE CONTRACT

For a contract to be enforced by the courts, certain elements must exist, as follows.[1]

1. There must be a *meeting of the minds* between the parties.
2. The subject of the contract must be a *legal subject*.
3. There must be *an offer and an acceptance*.
4. The contract must involve some *consideration*.
5. The parties must have *legal capacity* to enter into a contract.
6. The *terms* of the contract must be sufficiently precise.

Meeting of the Minds

Meeting of the minds

First there must be an agreement — a meeting of the minds. In the treadmill example, the two parties could have been discussing treadmills in general. The party wanting the treadmill was thinking in terms of a test-grade treadmill to be used in his new wellness center. The party selling the treadmill was thinking of a treadmill that the average client would use in the wellness center for walking purposes only. When the two parties made the deal, they were not making the deal with the same piece of equipment in mind. There was no meeting of the minds — no true agreement. Therefore, no contract exists.

Legal Subject

The subject of the contract must be a legal subject. Drug dealers cannot sue one another for breach of contract. In some instances, though, an act that would generally be considered legal is illegal. Most states have laws requiring teachers in public schools to be certified or licensed. These laws usually extend to coaches in public schools. Anyone who coaches in the public schools must be a certified or licensed teacher. If an administrator in a school in such a state were to hire an unlicensed teacher to coach a sport on a part-time basis, would this be illegal?

According to state law, this would be illegal and, therefore, no contract would exist. If a dispute were to arise over the agreement as to period of employment, salary to be paid, the sport or sports to be coached, and so on, the court would decide that these issues were of no importance because a contract did not exist in the first place. Some states that had such laws have recently modified the laws to allow noncertified and nonlicensed teachers to coach in the public schools — at least at the assistant coach level. This has been done to meet the increasing need for coaches and to avoid the type of problems mentioned in this example. Many in the exercise-related professions see this as an unwise decision. It creates a situation in which less qualified persons are coaching young people, and thereby increasing the risks to participants. This, in turn, increases the liability for everyone involved. (See "Qualitative Supervision" in Chapter 16.)

Offer and Acceptance

For a contract to exist, one party must make an offer and the other party must accept the offer. In a sale-of-goods situation, if the seller makes an offer for a specific item at a specific price to be delivered by a specific date and the buyer says, "I accept that offer, but can you deliver the goods a month earlier," does an offer exists? The answer is "no." The buyer has not made an acceptance. She has made a *counteroffer*. She changed the seller's offer. The seller must now accept the counteroffer or suggest another date, or he might suggest another price because the earlier shipping date might entail increased costs. Or he might say that he could get other merchandise that he has in stock for the same price on the requested date but not the merchandise the buyer wants.

Offer and acceptance

Counteroffer

The seller does not want to obligate himself to a deadline he cannot meet, and the buyer does not want to obligate herself to paying for merchandise that will not arrive by the time it is needed. Nor does she want to accept merchandise she really does not want. When one party totally accepts the conditions the other party places on the agreement, an offer and acceptance are complete.

Contract law is often difficult to understand, and it frequently creates unexpected problems for one or both parties. Nowhere is this more true than in offer and acceptance. In the example above, if the buyer and seller finally come to an agreement on the price and date of shipment and then the seller ships the merchandise he has in stock rather than the merchandise the buyer wanted, has he breached the contract? This question has no "yes" or "no" answer. If the invoice sent with the merchandise clearly shows that the merchandise is not what the buyer ordered and the buyer accepts it and begins to use it, the buyer has, by her act or deed, accepted a new offer.

In essence, what has happened is that a new offer and acceptance have been made. The seller has made a new offer by sending different merchandise clearly indicating by description in the invoice that it is not what the buyer ordered, and the buyer has made an acceptance by her act of accepting and using the merchandise rather than rejecting the shipment. The buyer is now required to meet her obligation under this new agreement, which is to pay the agreed-upon price as noted on the invoice or included in a separate bill that might arrive after the merchandise. This situation happens more often than we like to admit, especially in situations where the person receiving and distributing goods for use is not the person who ordered the goods.

When the parties start adding *contingencies*, or conditions, to their agreement, they are asking for even more problems. When one party makes an offer, the other party might counteroffer by placing on that offer a condition that will occur at a later date and the other party accepts that condition. If something happens to postpone the occurrence of the condition, is there still a contract? Maybe, or maybe not. Questions now must be answered as to *reasonableness*. Was placing the condition on the contract in the first place reasonable? Would a reasonable person anticipate postponements of the type that occurred? Was the time period in which the condition was to occur a reasonable period to wait, and has the postponement taken the time period beyond a reasonable waiting period?

Other questions are also likely to be raised. Was the accepting party under any pressure to accept the conditions? Did one party hold any undue influence over the other party that affected the offer or acceptance? It is not within the scope of this text to answer these questions. Nevertheless, consider these questions and the obvious difficulty in answering them as a word of warning to the wise. Keep the offer and acceptance as simple and to the point as possible, and include any contingencies only when absolutely necessary, assuring as much as possible that the conditions will occur.

Other questions concerning offer and acceptance can also arise. These are delineated as follows.[2]

1. *Are catalogs offers from a company?* The answer is "no." Catalogs are invitations to the buyer to make an offer to the seller by filling out the order form and sending it to the seller. Suppose the price for a piece of equipment in the catalog is printed incorrectly or the prices have

changed for some reason. Is the seller obligated to meet the price in the catalog? The answer is "no" because the catalog does not constitute an offer.

2. *How long is an offer effective?* Unless the offerer specifies a time for which the offer is good, the offer stands for a reasonable time and can be accepted any time during that reasonable period. If the offerer decides to withdraw the offer prior to an acceptance, he or she can do so, but only by informing the potential acceptor of the withdrawal.

3. *Does the use of unsolicited goods constitute an acceptance and thus obligate the user to pay for the goods?* The answer is "no." This is an age-old device that sellers use to make the receiver feel obligated to pay for the merchandise — usually because of guilt. Even though this practice is not used now as much as it was in the past, it still happens. Companies send "gifts" to potential buyers in hopes of getting their business. When the business is not forthcoming, some companies send a bill for the "gift." Since there is no offer and acceptance associated with this merchandise (and no meeting of the minds), there is no contract and no obligation on the receiver's part. Persons who feel guilty about receiving and not paying for this merchandise should return the merchandise unused. Most management texts recommend, concerning purchasing goods, never to accept gifts from sellers even though you are not obligated to pay for them.

4. *Are "free trial" offers treated the same as gifts sent by sellers?* Generally, no. Most free-trial offers that sellers make are for a given period, say 30 days, after which the full price of the merchandise is expected to be paid if the merchandise is retained. Most sellers ask the potential buyer to accept this offer by requesting the free trial. If potential buyers accept this offer, send for and receive the merchandise, and then let it sit on a shelf for 2 months, they are now obligated to pay the seller the full price whether they have any use for the merchandise or not.

Consideration

If there is to be an agreement between two parties, there must be an exchange of, or at least a promise of an exchange of, something of value between the two parties. The seller offers merchandise in exchange for money, or the promise to pay, from the buyer. The employer contracts to pay a salary and benefits in exchange for time and services from an employee.

Consideration

A buyer and a seller have an agreement, a contract, in which the seller is to send 12 dozen tennis balls to the buyer for $65.00 plus shipping and handling. The buyer receives the tennis balls and then decides not to make the payment. Can the buyer say she does not owe the amount due because a contract did not exist without consideration, or payment? Obviously not.

The contract was made (assuming that all other elements are present) when there was a promise to pay. If the buyer does not pay now, she will be in breach of a valid contract and the seller can take steps to make her pay.

Legal Capacity

Legal capacity

Legal capacity refers to an individual's age or mental capacity. Contracts made with minors, individuals with mental retardation, insane persons, or persons suffering from any type of mental incapacity are considered void-able contracts. This means that the minor or mentally incapacitated person can void the contract. The party making the contract with the minor or mentally incapacitated person, however, cannot void the contract. We

Void contract
Voidable contract

must be aware of the difference between a *void* contract and a *voidable* contract. If any of the other elements discussed here are missing, the contract is considered void and cannot be enforced. If all of the elements discussed above are present and the contract is made with a minor by an adult who has no mental incapacity, the minor can enforce the contract against the adult, but because the contract is voidable by the minor, the adult cannot enforce the contract against the minor if the minor decides not to abide by the terms of the contract.

Many exercise-related professionals deal with minors and mentally incapacitated persons regularly in athletic, recreational, and therapeutic situations. Problems of voidable contracts can be avoided by making any necessary contracts with the parents or guardians of these individuals.

Specificity of Terms

Specificity (of contractual terms)

Specificity of terms is a little different from the first five elements discussed. If the parties making a contract do not state the terms of the contract precisely concerning price, quantity, or payment and a dispute arises over the contract, a court will decide whether a contract exists or not based on what would be most fair to the parties involved. If the contract involves merchandise that has not been used and can be easily returned by the buyer and resold by the seller, the court is likely to find the contract void because of lack of specificity, and require the goods to be returned.

But what if the goods have been used already and the seller is demanding immediate payment and the buyer is saying that he has 6 months to pay? The court is not going to find the contract void because returning the used merchandise to the seller would be unfair. The court would review the contract and hear testimony from the two parties in an attempt to find the source of the disagreement. Whether the court finds the precise problem or not, it will make a decision that is as fair as possible to the two parties.

If the above example involves a relatively modest payment, the buyer will most likely be able to make the payment regardless of the length of time the court decides. If a large sum is involved, however, or if interest rates or shipping and handling payments significantly alter what the buyer was expecting to pay or the seller was expecting to receive, the court's decision could be devastating to one of the parties.

The same is true in contracts of employment or personal services. This type of contract can easily be vague. This creates a situation in which one or both parties are likely to be disappointed in what is received from the other party. Often these disappointments are not realized until well into the contract period, when an employee is told that her contract will not be renewed because she has not performed as expected or an employee sues for a benefit that supposedly was to be included but was not.

The only way to overcome the problems of specificity is to be as detailed as possible when negotiating the terms of any contract. This is important in any contract and particularly important in contracts dealing with large sums of money and with employment contracts. It is not a bad idea to have such contracts reviewed by a lawyer before finalizing them. If you were to take a job that required you to sign a contract, what would you want included in that contract and how would you expect a potential employer to negotiate your desired terms?

BREACH OF CONTRACT

In the discussion above, the term *breach* was used frequently. Breach of contract means that one of the parties has failed to meet his obligation created by the agreement. For a breach to occur, there must be a contract. All of the elements of a contract must be met. If they are not, the contract is void, and a void contract cannot be breached because there is no contract in the first place. If one party breaches a contract, he cannot in turn claim that the other party has breached the contract. If the seller and the buyer have an enforceable contract and the seller ships the wrong merchandise, the seller has breached the contract. He cannot then claim that the buyer has breached the contract by not sending a payment.

The same is true for personal service contracts. Someone seeking your services as a physical therapist might agree to pay you a specified amount prior to your beginning the service and then so much each week or month as the service is delivered. The party cannot claim a breach on your part for not delivering the service when you do not deliver because you have not received the initial payment. The person has already breached.

Breaches can be either immaterial or material. *Immaterial breaches* are not likely to cause the rest of the contract to fail. They might be

Immaterial breach of contract

disconcerting and cause you to have questions about the party with which you are dealing, but they should not cause lawsuits. Immaterial breaches should be worked out between the parties. This does not mean that one of the parties has not experienced some loss, but it would generally be less than what would be involved in going to court.

For example, a buyer and a seller agree on a certain shipping date and a certain mode of shipment. The seller is to pay the shipping costs. The seller is late in getting the shipment together and, to meet the shipping date, has to use a different mode of shipping. This causes an increase in the shipment cost, and the seller, rather than incurring the cost himself, adds the difference between the original shipping cost and the actual shipping cost to the buyer's bill.

Is the buyer obligated to pay this additional cost? Only if the contract had some agreement stating that the buyer would pay any shipping cost above a specified amount. Otherwise, the seller has breached the contract. Because this is immaterial to the overall contract, the buyer should send a check for the agreed-upon cost, which does not include the extra shipping cost. If the seller wants to sue, that is up to him, but he will not win and will have to pay his and possibly the buyer's court cost.

Material breach of contract

Material breaches are another story. They relieve the nonbreaching party of any obligations imposed by the contract. Material breaches indicate that one of the parties has or has not done something that significantly affects the other party. If the breaching party is not willing to correct the problem, material breaches will generally be settled in court.

Material breaches are often tied to the specificity of terms of the contract. What one party sees as being material might not be seen as material by the other party. If the buyer wants specific merchandise by a specific date, how does she ensure that the seller knows this date is material to the contract? The buyer must state that *time is of the essence*. If the buyer wants to ensure that the seller does not send equipment that is below standard, she must *list specifications in detail*. If the seller then is late in shipping the merchandise or ships substandard equipment, he has materially breached the contract and has no excuse for not knowing that these were material considerations. These are only two examples of specificity of terms that can indicate the materiality of various considerations. There are many other ways in which specificity of terms can affect materiality, depending on the nature of the contract.

Specific performance

If a contract is breached, the nonbreaching party can sue for damages, usually in the form of money, or for *specific performance*. If the nonbreaching party still wants the contract to be fulfilled because she can still use the goods or services and no other goods or services will suffice, she will typically sue for specific performance. This means just what it appears to mean. The nonbreacher wants the breaching party to perform specifically as indicated in the original agreement. If the court believes specific performance is equitable, the court will order the breaching party to meet the specific obligations of the contract.

If specific performance is no longer possible or the nonbreaching party wants specific performance, the nonbreaching party will sue for damages. Sometimes determining whether any damages exist is difficult. Say an athletic director orders new uniforms for the football team and the uniforms are to be delivered 1 month before the season begins. The day the uniforms are to be delivered, the athletic director receives a call informing him that the company cannot deliver the uniforms — not only on the agreed upon date, but not at all. If the athletic director cannot find another company to furnish the same quality of uniforms for the same price by the time the uniforms are needed, does he suffer any damage?

Several fitness experts are opening a new fitness center and have ordered a large quantity of free weights and weight machines for their weight room. A week before delivery is due, they receive a call informing them that the equipment will be several months late. This date is 1 month after the center is to open. They have already sold a large number of memberships. Many of the persons buying these memberships did so specifically because they were excited about having such a well-equipped weight facility in their neighborhood. Many of these memberships likely will be lost if the equipment is not there on opening day. Have the buyers experienced damage? Consider this situation and the one above, and determine whether you believe damages exist or not and, if so, to what money damages the nonbreaching party might be entitled.

One way to avoid having to determine money damages after the fact is to consider these beforehand and include in the agreement a *liquidated damages clause*. Liquidated damages require the parties to anticipate certain problems and set an amount that must be paid if those problems do arise and create a material breach. If there is a material breach, the breaching party is obligated to pay the agreed-upon amount stated in the

Liquidated damages

liquidated damages clause. The amount agreed upon should be as close as possible to the actual damages that would result from a breach. Liquidated damages should serve as encouragement, but not punishment, for both parties to meet their obligations. The courts typically will not uphold liquidated damage amounts that are exorbitant.

The comments above apply to contracts for the purchase of goods and for personal service. The two types of contracts, however, do have some differences that are unique to each.

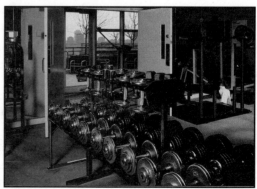

Free weight room.

PURCHASE OF GOODS AND THE UNIFORM COMMERCIAL CODE

Caveat emptor

For many years, the phrase *caveat emptor* controlled the purchase of goods. It means, "Let the buyer beware." Basically buyers were responsible for ensuring that what they saw was actually what they thought they saw. If someone purchased a bottle of Mama's Elixir from a traveling salesman who promised that the potion would relieve everything from arthritis to urinary track infections, she had no recourse when she discovered that the potion was nothing more than watered-down maple syrup.

Caveat vendor

Even though the buyer should still beware, some of the responsibility for ensuring that buyers are getting what they expect has now been shifted to the sellers. The phrase *caveat vendor*, or "Let the seller beware," is a reality because of the requirements of the Uniform Commercial Code (UCC). All jurisdictions in the United States have adopted the UCC or some portions of it as a means of providing fairness in dealings between the buyers and the sellers of goods. The two provisions of the UCC that are most likely to protect the buyer beyond the protections of the agreement made with the seller are the *implied warranty of merchantability* and the *implied warranty of fitness for a particular use*.

Implied Warranty of Merchantability

Implied warranty of merchantability

An *implied warranty* means that buyers automatically expect the goods they purchase to be warranted. There need be nothing in writing from the seller telling the buyer that this particular warranty is in effect. And what does it mean to have a warranty of merchantability that is automatically in effect? According to the UCC, it means that the item sold to the purchaser is at least of the general kind described and is reasonably fit for the general purpose for which it was sold. The seller is expected to sell what she has described to the buyer, and when the buyer receives the goods, he will be able to use them under normal conditions for the expected purpose without their falling apart.

Two elements must be present for this warranty to be in effect:

1. The goods must be purchased from a merchant who deals in that type of goods.

2. The goods must fall below the minimum quality acceptable in the trade for that type of goods.

The first element alerts buyers to purchase goods only from dealers that typically deal in the goods purchased. This means you should not buy a whirlpool for your training room from a dealer who typically sells athletic tape. The second element is simply the condition necessary for triggering the warranty. If the goods you purchase are not below the minimum quality acceptable, you do not have to be concerned with the warranty in the first place.

Implied Warranty of Fitness for a Particular Purpose

Implied warranty of fitness

The implied warranty of fitness for a particular use provides that, if an item that is sold is ordinarily used in but one way, its fitness for use in that specific way is impliedly warranted unless there is evidence to the contrary. For this warranty to be in effect, (1) the goods must be purchased from a merchant who deals in that type of goods, (2) at the time of sale, the seller must have reason to know that the buyer was going to use the product for a particular use, and (3) the buyer was relying on the seller's skill or judgment to select or furnish suitable goods for that particular purpose.

These elements are self-explanatory and show that this warranty is not as automatic as the implied warranty of merchantability. This warranty comes into effect when the buyer is seeking advice from the seller on goods used in specific situations and makes clear to the buyer that this equipment is to be used for a particular purpose, not just general use. Once the seller accepts this role and recommends the goods for this particular purpose, this warranty comes into effect.

Persons responsible for ordering supplies and equipment for exercise-related programs should be aware of these two warranties. If all elements of a contract for the sale of goods seem to have been met, yet the goods delivered fail when used or cannot be used as expected, these two warranties allow the buyer to return the goods, even after they are used, for a refund or a replacement. If the seller fails to provide a replacement or give a refund, the buyer can sue using the appropriate warranty as the basis of the suit.

CONTRACTS FOR PERSONAL SERVICES

Contracts for personal services are typically agreements between an individual employer and the individual whose services are being sought or between an employer, or the employer's negotiators, and a designated group of employees representing all other employees. The latter case is typical when unions have a bargaining group that negotiates a contract. In this case, people seeking employment either accept the contract and provide the services or look elsewhere for employment if they do not like the contract.

The advantage of such a contract is that persons working in the particular environment are familiar with the conditions and with what they think is fair exchange for their services. Their experience helps ensure that all the appropriate elements of the contract are present, especially in relation to the preciseness of the terms of the contract. They ensure that all benefits are included and that conditions concerning evaluation, remediation, and termination are stated clearly. Such organizations generally have the assistance of legal counsel in formulating the agreement. Of course, the disadvantage of this contract is that no single employee or potential employee has any individual bargaining power.

If an individual wants such bargaining power, he should seek out situations in which he can negotiate his contract individually. When negotiating an individual contract, the elements of an enforceable contract must be kept in mind. In addition, the individual should be aware of the status of employment. An individual being hired by an employer typically is hired as a part-time employee, a full-time employee, or an *independent contractor.*

Independent contractor

Coaches, personal trainers, therapists, athletic trainers, and the like might find themselves in a position to be hired as independent contractors. Although this might sound attractive, it is desirable only when the service provider wishes to maintain her independence. If an employer needs a service for a specified time only, he is likely to make an agreement with the service provider as an independent contractor. This means the employer is not responsible for paying income taxes, social security, or worker compensation for the independent contractor. The independent contractor is responsible for paying these, and for the bookkeeping necessary for doing so.

The employer is also not responsible for the acts of the independent contractor. The legal concept of *respondeat superior* does not apply in cases where the relationship is one of employer and independent contractor. The employer does not have to answer for the negligence of the independent contractor. Also, *hold-harmless* laws that apply to most public institutions do not apply to independent contractors. These laws allow for the protection and defense of an employee who is acting on behalf of the employer by the employer. Because the independent contractor is not an employee in the strict definition of the term, the employer cannot defend her. The independent contractor is not eligible for any benefits from the employer. The employer generally prefers these conditions. The employee may not.

Like the independent contractor, the part-time employee is typically not eligible for most benefits from the employer. That is where the comparison ends. The employer is responsible for withholding income taxes, paying its share of social security taxes, and paying unemployment and/or worker compensation insurance premiums. In some situations, the individual who is seeking part-time employment can negotiate for benefits from the employer, so this should not be ignored.

Full-time employees are eligible for benefits from the employer. In situations where the benefits might vary and are not some set package provided to all full-time employees, the individual negotiating with the employer should ensure that he negotiates for the benefit package that best suits his needs.

These are not the only considerations to be included in a contract. We will not go into the details of individual contract negotiations here. People who negotiate their own contracts should seek legal assistance in reviewing an agreement to ensure that all bases are covered. Some contracts, especially those for higher-level positions, can be quite complicated.

Contracts between an employer and an employee are generally for a set period of time. The contract typically indicates the period for which the contract is valid. It is also reasonable to include, in the contract, conditions under which the contract will be terminated if the terms of the contract are not completed. We often wonder why a coach who has a 5-year contract with school A can leave after 3 years to take a position with school B. This is generally possible because both the coach and school A provided for this in the conditions for termination, and they are simply following through on their agreement. If either party breaches the contract, the other party is not responsible for meeting its obligations created by the agreement.

In Chapter 14, we noted that people employed by governmental entities could not be deprived of their property interest without due process of law. Where a property right has been created and the employee has not breached the terms of employment outright, the governmental employer cannot take the property right away without giving cause. This right exists whether a contract does or does not exist.

In the area of private employment, a contract provides similar protection for the employee. If an employer releases an employee who has met the terms of the contract prior to the end of the contract for no valid reason, the employer can be charged with breach of contract and the released employee can sue the employer for damages. Of course, the private employer can have the same reasons of cause as would a public employer for releasing an employee prior to the end of a contract.

Valid causes for termination of employment are known as the three I's:

1. *Immorality* (e.g., dishonesty, theft, lying, sexual misconduct)

2. *Insubordination* (e.g., continually arguing with a supervisor in such a way that the program is affected, refusing to attend required meetings, ignoring instructions from a supervisor, failing to adhere to established policies)

3. *Incompetence* (e.g., lack of knowledge of the job, failure to exercise sufficient supervision, not fulfilling the duties of the job in a professional manner).

To be considered as just cause for terminating a contract, any of these examples must occur in connection with the job. Immorality in one's private life, for example, might be deplorable, but if it is not in any way connected to the job or if it is not having any effect on the job, it is not a valid reason for dismissal.

Suffice it to say that in contracts for either goods or personal services, one should ensure that all elements of the contract are present, it is in writing, liquidated damages clauses are considered, and all terms of performance significant to both parties, including conditions of termination, are included.

NOTES

1. L. J. Carpenter. *Legal Concepts in Sport: A Primer* (Reston, VA: American Alliance for Health, Physical Education, Recreation and Dance, 1995).

2. Carpenter.

RESOURCES

Appenzeller, H. Employment of coaches: Is the right to hire the right to fire?. In *Sports and Law: Contemporary Issues*, edited by H. Appenzeller (1985). Charlottesville, VA: Michie Co.

Dougherty, N. J., et al (1994). *Sport, Physical Activity, and the Law*. Champaign, IL: Human Kinetics.

Nolan, J. R., and J. M. Nolan-Haley, (1990). *Black's Law Dictionary*, 6th ed. St. Paul: West Publishing.

Risk Management

OBJECTIVES

After studying this chapter, you should be able to:

1. Define risk management.
2. Discuss how risk management is part of the ongoing process of planning and presenting programs.
3. Define standard of care and list and discuss factors within a program that will affect the standard of care expected in that program.
4. Identify the three areas in which most injuries occur in exercise-related programs, and give examples of the types of injuries that are most likely in each area.
5. Define qualitative and quantitative supervision and specific and general supervision.
6. Discuss at least five ways to improve the effectiveness of supervision.
7. Discuss at least five ways to assure proper selection and conduct of activities.
8. Outline a procedure for inspecting facilities and equipment and for remedying any problems found.
9. Discuss at least five ways to ensure safe environmental conditions.
10. Give an example of each of the three ways that risks can be transferred.
11. Give at least two examples of state statutes that might transfer liability for the exercise-related professional.

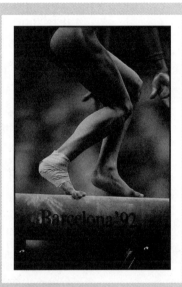

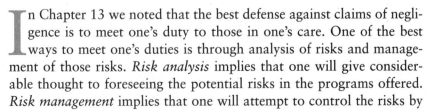

In Chapter 13 we noted that the best defense against claims of negligence is to meet one's duty to those in one's care. One of the best ways to meet one's duties is through analysis of risks and management of those risks. *Risk analysis* implies that one will give considerable thought to foreseeing the potential risks in the programs offered. *Risk management* implies that one will attempt to control the risks by

Risk analysis
Risk
management

removing them, or controlling those that cannot be removed, or possibly transferring the liability for the risks to others.

Attention to risks is a never-ending task in the exercise-related professions. It begins long before participation in a program ever starts. Risk management begins in initial program planning when the types of programs are being chosen. Programs typically are selected to meet the needs or desires of specific groups. Society is demanding more active and higher risk activities over a wider range of ages. This creates a demand for better-trained instructors and improved facilities that can offer a variety of activities.

If facilities and personnel are available already, the programs selected must be appropriate for those personnel and facilities. If a specific program is desired and appropriate facilities and personnel are not available, personnel (for both instruction and management) must be selected and facilities must be developed to meet the specific needs of the desired program.

Once programs have been selected, risk management continues with the specific elements of pre-program administration. Daily program plans and objectives related to specific age groups, ability levels, and disabilities must be developed in relation to the nature of the activity. Policies must be formulated for dealing with risks that cannot be removed. Policies must be written concerning daily inspections, reporting discrepancies found, and steps necessary for adequate follow-up. Procedures must be made for dealing with emergency situations and for reporting those situations. And all personnel must be made aware of and know how to implement these policies and procedures.

Once program presentation begins, risk management shifts to (1) proper supervision and (2) conduct of activities in (3) an environment conducive to safe implementation of the program. In addition to the actual act of conducting the activity for the participants, the program provider must be continuously aware of the risks associated with these three aspects of program presentation. Whether one meets her obligations for the care of those in her programs or does not meet her obligations in these three areas determines whether or not she meets her standard of care.

STANDARD OF CARE

When a program provider acts as a risk manager, he is attempting to meet his duty of care to those in his programs. This duty of care arises out of the relationship between the professional and those participating in his programs. Case law or precedent has established this duty. Nothing need be signed between the program provider and the participant to establish this duty. The level of the duty the program provider is to exhibit is called the *standard of care*.

Standard of care

The standard of care that the professional must exhibit to meet his duty arises out of the concept of reasonableness and will vary from situation to situation. If a parent leaves her child in the care of someone who is providing a program for that child, the parent expects that the program provider will care for this child at least at the level expected of a reasonable parent. If the program provided is merely one of supervision and daily care of the child's needs, this standard of care may be sufficient. If, however, this program involves some type of instruction and training or some type of rehabilitative protocol, the standard of care rises. The standard of care is now the minimum level expected of a reasonable professional providing that service. And the ability to foresee risks associated with one's program is part of that minimum expectancy.

The standard of care must be sufficient to protect the participant from the foreseeable risk of unreasonable harm.[1] The responsibility to meet and the ability of the professional to meet, this standard will not only vary according to the services provided but also will depend upon a host of factors based on the nature of the setting. The following factors will vary in any given circumstance and, therefore, affect the standard of care expected:[2]

- age and maturity of participants
- skill of participants
- health and conditioning status of participants
- size of group involved
- complexity of the program
- hazardous nature of the program
- age, skill, and size of the competitors (in contact activities)
- amount of supervision present
- significance of safety hazards present because of facilities or equipment
- atmosphere/logistics/nature of the area in which the activity will take place (visibility, traffic, time of day, criminal element)
- accessibility of medical assistance.

These factors affect the standard of care required individually and in combination. The likelihood of accidents goes up as the number of participants goes up and the skill level of the participants goes down. In this situation, one must anticipate the need for closer supervision and more direct instruction. If, however, only one person is available to supervise an increasing number of unskilled participants, that one person will likely not be able to meet the standard of care necessary for the group. Therefore, the size of the group must be limited or more instructors must be provided. If this is not done and an injury occurs, those providing the program will be negligent and will be liable — even for injuries that were inherent in the activity — because they did not meet their standard of care. Anticipating this potential problem through risk management is no guarantee against injuries. Taking heed of potential problems and making appropriate alterations to the program, however, are indications that the program providers were making every attempt to meet their standard of care.

When program providers fail to manage the risks associated with the above factors, injuries are likely to occur and lawsuits are apt to be brought against the program providers. A survey of 1994 lawsuits indicates that most of the injuries for which lawsuits are brought are caused by one of the following:

1. Faulty supervision.

2. Inappropriate selection or conduct of activities.

3. Unsafe environmental conditions.[3]

Often, risk management is thought of only in terms of providing a safe environment. Management of the risks in supervision and selection and conduct of activities is equally critical in meeting one's standard of care to participants. An examination of these areas will help to identify the types of risks associated with each area.

Supervision

Qualitative supervision

Adequate supervision is related to both the quality of the supervision given, *qualitative supervision,* and the supervisor/participant ratio, *quantitative supervision.* Qualitative supervision is related to the training of the individuals who provide the program of activities. This aspect of supervision is important to the persons directly responsible for providing supervision to the participants, as well as to persons at higher administrative levels who are indirectly responsible for this supervision. Upon taking a position of employment, those directly responsible for supervision are expected to meet the minimum standards for their profession. They are also expected to keep their training current by attending workshops and seminars, reading current literature, and updating certifications as needed.

Respondeat superior

Persons in higher administrative positions are also liable for this type of supervision through the civil-law concept of *respondeat superior.* This literally means, "Let the master answer." The administrators, the masters, are expected to provide program providers who are qualified to appropriately supervise others. They are also responsible for qualitative supervision themselves. They are responsible for ensuring that their employees are up to date in their training and certifications. They are responsible for evaluating their employees, determining if deficiencies exist, and providing plans to correct any existing deficiencies.

If program participants incur injuries because of inadequacies of the employees over whom the administrators have control, the administrators are *vicariously liable* through the actions of the employees even though the administrator had no direct control over the activity in which the injury occurred. Administrators can also be charged directly for *negligent hiring*. Administrators must assure that the credentials of the persons they hire are valid. In today's world, administrators also have to check into the backgrounds of potential employees. This is of special importance when the employee will be working with children. Even though this is a recent concern in employment and has yet to be fully litigated in the courts, employers should be advised to be diligent in this area.

It is foreseeable that injuries are likely to occur as a result of shortcomings in qualitative supervision by the instructor and the instructor's superiors. Proper risk management would tell us not to hire personnel who are not qualified to perform the tasks for which they are hired. Proper risk management would tell us to ensure that personnel are kept up-to-date as techniques and methodologies change and as new equipment and technologies are introduced. Even though we are most likely to meet the foreseeable risks by hiring qualified personnel and updating the personnel already on staff, we also meet these foreseeable risks by passing them on. Passing on the risk will be discussed later.

Quantitative supervision is related to the number of participants in a program in relation to the number of persons needed for adequate supervision. This is not a simple ratio of 20:1 or any other such ratio. The appropriate number of supervisors is determined by the nature of the activity and the conditions under which the activity is provided.

Quantitative supervision

For example, with certain types of injuries, a therapist might have to work one-on-one with her client. Sharing her time with another client would jeopardize the safety of the client who needs her constant attention. In other situations, the therapists might rotate among several clients during the same time period without diminishing the care given. In either case, the ratio of participants to supervisors is relatively low. Even when supervising more than one client, the therapist should have little difficulty maintaining contact with each. If something happens with one client that demands more attention than planned, though, supervision of the other clients will likely be decreased. This is a situation in which *general supervision* is interrupted by the need for *specific supervision*. In a clinical situation, interruptions are foreseeable and can be handled by calling on other therapists to assist in supervising clients who need only general supervision.

General supervision Specific supervision

Good planning as a result of risk analysis prepares people in the situation described above to react to the needs of one another. They anticipate these occurrences because they have foreseen and discussed the likelihood of the situation. They will have a plan of action to put into place. Poor planning and no risk analysis will result in confusion at the time of emergency and a likely lack of supervision to all clients. This type of break in supervision is what results in the faulty supervision that causes injuries.

In situations where only one supervisor is present, such as teaching a large physical education class or working with a large group in a wellness setting, the need for specific supervision arises often, with little likelihood that anyone will be there to assist. When the teacher must give specific instruction to a student who is having difficulty, he can never forget to maintain general supervision of the other students in the class. He must be constantly aware of what is taking place and what others in the class are likely to be doing. This is especially true if equipment that is being used presents a danger when not appropriately supervised or if participants are beginners and might attempt activities that are above their capabilities while they are not being watched.

The following guidelines increase the effectiveness of supervision:[4]

- Take all reasonable steps to keep supervisory/instructional skills and certifications at the highest possible level.
- Organize the participants to facilitate effective supervision.
- Do not leave individuals or groups unsupervised.
- Establish, post, explain, and enforce general behavioral and safety rules for all areas.
- Secure facilities and equipment not being used.
- Be prepared to render immediate and effective first aid when necessary.
- Develop emergency procedures to be followed in the event of an accident or injury.
- Keep in mind that supervisors must maintain control of their participants at all time.

If these guidelines are undertaken with the realization that when they are not accomplished, the risks to participants in the program increases, personnel will be more likely to see the need for, and accept, what they must do.

Selection and Conduct of Activities

The activities used in any program must match the participants' ability and characteristics. A teacher or a coach who selects skills for students and athletes who have not been properly trained for those activities violates this crucial guideline. The same is true for an exercise leader who prescribes exercise that is too strenuous for her participants in a fitness club or corporate wellness setting and for the athletic trainer who recommends an activity for an athlete who is not ready to move to an advanced level because of a previous injury.

The provider of the activity must be aware of the status of the participant at all times and foresee the potential for risks of improperly selected activities. In addition to risk analysis, this requires regular assessment of the participants before and during participation. This will involve skill tests, fitness tests, medical examinations, and the like to establish readiness and ability to participate in a given activity. It will involve the use of appropriate lead-up activities and protocols to assure that participants who are behind have the opportunity to advance their skill level or regain skills lost as a result of injury or disuse.

Further, the provider of the activity must remember that readiness to participate applies to each individual participant and not to some group average. Even if the majority of participants in a group are ready to go to higher-level participation, some of the participants may not be ready to move on. The teacher or coach must recognize the need for more individual attention or practice time for some students and athletes. The exercise leader must be aware that some participants need more time to improve their strength and fitness at one level before advancing to the next. The athletic trainer and therapist must be constantly alert to the reality that some of their athletes/patients will not respond to therapy as expected and, therefore, will need more time than recommended for a specific protocol.

Once an activity provider thinks she has selected the appropriate activities for her participants, she must ensure that the conduct of the activity is also appropriate. The provider must have a well-established plan for presenting the activity. This plan must be in writing with appropriate goals and objectives to be accomplished and must include methodologies appropriate for attaining the objectives. (Doing things during the presentation of an activity that have no relation to objectives to be accomplished means that plans are not being followed. This increases the likelihood of mistakes that can lead to injuries.) There must also be statements indicating alternative methods for participants who are not progressing as expected, as well as alternative plans to be followed when adjustments are needed because of interruptions in the program.

Teachers will recognize this as the unit-planning process with daily lesson plans. Coaches will recognize this as their coaching plan for the progression of a team over a season. Trainers and therapists will recognize this as the protocol for dealing with a specific injury or a class of injuries (for both prevention and rehabilitation). Exercise/wellness specialists will recognize this as their program design for intervening with specific lifestyle components to improve the participants' health status. These professionals should also recognize that all of these plans are based not only on a purpose of teaching a certain skill or overcoming a specific injury but also for the purpose of progressively moving a participant from one point to another as efficiently as possible. Foreseeability of potential risks guides us to do only that which the participant is capable of doing.

Regardless of the provider, the methods used to attain the objectives set for the program must include instruction that participants can easily understand. Participants must clearly know what they are to accomplish. They must understand that they are at point A and are expected to move to point B by following steps 1, 2, 3, 4, and so forth, which the program provider has laid out. Participants also must know that this procedure is expected to take a given amount of time, but some will be accelerated and some may lag behind. The participants should also know that assessment will be used along the way to provide feedback to the provider so the amount of progress toward the objectives for the activity can be determined. The provider must be aware that simply giving what she believes is adequate instruction is not enough. Feedback indicating that the instructions are being followed and progress is being made is a necessity for meeting the standard of care in this area.

Instruction also must include warnings of any potential hazards inherent to the activity in which the participants are to be involved. Risk analysis puts us on the alert that every hazard cannot be removed from many of the activities we offer, particularly those in which participants are moving and are likely to come in contact with one another or with objects in the environment. In addition to warnings of the hazards, participants should be given instructions to minimize the risks associated with the hazards. These instructions should be incorporated into the plan for the activities. They may be given at the beginning of instruction as a specific warning and then reiterated as part of the actual step-by-step procedure of presenting the activity.

Football provides an excellent example. Prior to beginning practice at any level, a coach will warn his players of potential risks inherent in the game, particularly those that might occur if the players fail to follow the directions the coaches give. During this time, specific warnings are given concerning the devastating effects of head and neck injuries resulting from improper tackling techniques. This warning will be followed by instruction, at the appropriate time, on proper tackling techniques, during which a description of improper tackling techniques and their inherent risks will also be presented. A written plan showing this process followed by the actual presentations addresses this standard of care.

The following guidelines are offered for the selection and conduct of activities:[5]

■ Utilize or allow only activities that are within the participants' reasonable ability levels.

- Implement and document screening and pretesting procedures, and provide individualized progressions and lead-ups.

- Thoroughly plan presentations written such that they provide documentary evidence of sequential learning experiences, attention to critical safety factors, and organizational details, as well as the nature and extent of warnings provided.

- Ensure that all activities planned contribute to the objectives of the program.

- Prepare alternative plans for activities that are subject to frequent uncontrollable modifications.

- Develop routine procedures for excusing participants for medical complaints or injuries and for resuming participation following an injury or illness.

- Do not force participants to participate if they express strong fear, insecurity, or reluctance to participate.

- Provide any and all protective measures and devices appropriate to the activity, and require their routine use.

- In contact activities, carefully organize the group to reduce the likelihood and extent of mismatch situations.

- Carefully examine all elements of the program, take all reasonable steps to remove or control the identifiable risks, and make a conscious judgment as to whether the value of the activity significantly outweighs the risks that remain.

Safe Environmental Conditions

Ensuring that facilities and equipment are safe for use and are used safely are standard duties for all who offer activities. Whether the activity is a therapeutic treatment in a whirlpool or instruction on a climbing wall in a fitness center, program providers are expected to know of unsafe conditions in their facilities and of detectable defects in their equipment. Because unsafe conditions and defective equipment are foreseeable risks, policies and procedures must be in place to regularly inspect the facilities and equipment. Procedures should outline how to carry out the check — what to look for and the act of completing the appropriate paperwork. Policies should establish who will check what facilities and equipment, when they will be checked, for what purpose they are being checked, how reports are filed, and who must be notified when deficiencies are found.

An important part of the policy related to inspection of equipment and facilities is what is to be done when deficiencies are found. If the person performing the inspection can easily correct the condition, the policy should direct him to do so. If the condition can be corrected only by someone from a maintenance staff or from an outside service source, the policy should include procedures for putting the affected area or equipment off limits.

If equipment is defective, isolating the equipment or rendering it totally inoperable will keep others from using it. To isolate a facility or an area is not as easy. Program providers typically want to continue to use the area, especially if some time will pass before a condition is repaired. In most cases, an area can continue to be used as long as the participants are made aware of any existing hazard, receive instruction on how to avoid the hazard, and the program is modified to bring the affected area into play as little as possible.

Policies also should ensure that appropriate records are kept showing who was notified of the need for repair of a defect and what was needed. The records also should indicate a response from the persons notified with some indication of the time the repair is expected. This provides a basis for follow-up if the repair is taking longer than expected.

When dealing with maintenance staffs in-house, using triplicate work order forms is a good idea. This allows one copy to be kept with the originator of the work order and the other two to be sent to maintenance. When maintenance completes the repair, the repairer indicates on the work order the remedial action along with his signature and date. He retains a copy for the maintenance office and sends the final copy to the originator. The originator then has two copies on file, one showing the original request and its corresponding date and the second showing that the repair has been accomplished, by whom, and when.

Even though this notice to others might transfer some of the liability to those notified, it will not totally relieve of their liability those who found the defect and use the area or equipment on a regular basis. They maintain their responsibility to provide safe facilities and equipment for their participants as part of meeting their standard of care.

Actual notice

Program providers are said to have *actual notice* of defective conditions when they discover them or if others bring the problems to their attention. This expectation, however, goes beyond actual notice. Program providers also have *constructive notice* of such defects even if they do not inspect or hear of the defects from others. This is because they *should have known* about the defects because they should have done their inspection. Regardless of the type of notice, program providers are responsible for correcting any problems that exist, altering the program if the problem cannot be remedied, or giving appropriate warnings to participants to avoid an area or a piece of equipment.

Constructive notice

Program providers cannot expect to avoid fault when an injury is caused by a condition they could have corrected with a simple inspection.

A teacher who lets students participate on a field that has broken glass is likely to be held responsible for a child who is seriously cut while participating in a physical education activity. An athletic trainer could be at fault for injuries caused by frayed wires on a whirlpool. A therapist would be considered negligent if injury was caused by equipment that was not calibrated appropriately. The list goes on and on: if wet floors are not detected; if loose bolts are not tightened; if faulty protective equipment continues to be used. Vigilance in considering all potential problems and diligence in correcting or controlling all problems are the keys to meeting this standard of care.

The following guidelines will help program providers meet this standard of care:[6]

- Begin each day by inspecting the facilities and equipment to be used.

- If environmental hazards are detected but cannot be corrected immediately, take actions to isolate the area or equipment until repairs can be completed.

- Where appropriate, teach participants to perform basic safety inspections of the equipment they will be using and require them to do so as part of their daily routine. (This does not replace the program provider's duty to inspect the equipment, but it does increase the likelihood that existing defects will be found because more people are looking.)

- Do not allow running on slippery or uneven surfaces, and assure that participants are wearing the appropriate footwear for the activity in which they are participating.

- When selecting equipment or activity areas, make sure they meet or exceed applicable safety standards.

TRANSFERRING LIABILITY AS A MEANS OF RISK MANAGEMENT

Transferring one's liability appears to be a concept counter to what has already been presented concerning the duty of program presenters to participants. Because all risks in some programs cannot be removed and will continue to present problems for the program provider, it is preferable to ameliorate some of the liability to whatever extent possible. This transfer usually takes the form of (1) informing the participant of the risks, (2) contracting with the participant or others to transfer the risks, or (3) removing the liability altogether through State statute.

Transfer by informing the participant of the risks was mentioned in Chapter 13 as a defense to claims of negligence under the concept of *assumption of the risks*. In this case, liability for the risks is being transferred to the participant. The transfer is made by informing the adult participant of the risks and having him agree to accept these risks as an inherent part of the activity, usually by having the individual sign a *participation agreement* (see Appendix A.) Because the adult has a duty to self to act with care when participating in an activity that has risks, this transfer works. If the adult participant neglects this duty to self and is injured, the transfer is completed by holding the participant liable for his injuries through contributory negligence.

Contracting with the participant to transfer liability for risks takes several forms. The two most commonly used are the *release* and the *waiver*. These two are often considered to be the same, but nothing could be farther from the truth.

Waivers

Waivers are contracts signed by adult participants who are releasing their right to sue the program provider(s) for ordinary negligence that results in injury to the participant. (Such contracts cannot be enforced against minors, and adults cannot waive the rights of minors; therefore, waivers are valid only for adults.) Waivers do not cover gross negligence or intentional torts. Waiver contracts that include releases from gross negligence or intentional torts are typically considered void even though some jurisdictions will throw out the voiding language and keep only the language related to ordinary negligence. The waiver is one of the most direct means for transferring liability for risks. It is signed prior to participation and generally is accepted as long as it is written clearly and executed by adults who have comparable bargaining rights. *Comparable bargaining rights* means that the participant is under no pressure or inducement to sign the contract.

Releases

Whereas a waiver is signed before participation, a release is signed only after an injury has occurred during participation. A release is an agreement in which the injured party, who is an adult, agrees not to hold the program provider liable for injuries sustained in the program in exchange for some consideration, usually a sum of money, from the program provider. Unlike the waiver, the release is not a true transfer of liability at all. In essence, the program provider is admitting her liability and is hopefully limiting her losses by agreeing to pay a set sum of money.

Liability Insurance

The most common way to transfer liability to others (who are not participants) is through the purchase of insurance. *Professional liability insurance* is available through most professional organizations at a reasonable cost to the insured. The insurance will pay for expenses of a trial and judgments, up to the limits of the policy, against the insured should he lose the case. If the judgment exceeds the policy limits, the insured is liable for the excess. Professional liability insurance does not cover claims of gross negligence or intentional torts. Liability insurance covers only claims against ordinary negligence that occur in the performance of one's job.

Program providers should make sure that they know the details of their job description. Program providers often do things they think are an extension of their job only to find out that what they have done is an *ultra vires* activity — an activity performed without any authority to do so. If the activity is *ultra vires* and the program provider is negligent in performing that activity, neither the liability insurance he obtained through his professional organization nor the liability insurance his employer provides will cover any expenses if negligence claims are brought against him.

In some instances, an employer might provide liability insurance for employees. The policy limits, however, are generally low and are not likely to be enough to cover judgments in most negligence claims. Because of this, professionals are advised to have additional personal coverage.

Some states have enacted statutes that transfer liability under certain conditions. Some jurisdictions have *hold-harmless laws*, in which the State will defend certain groups of public employees against claims of ordinary negligence associated with the performance of their duties on the job. In some jurisdictions, public school teachers, coaches, and public recreation personnel are included in the group covered. If covered, there is no cost to the teacher, coach, or recreator for this defense. No such coverage exists for exercise-related professionals in the private sector.

Hold-harmless laws

Some jurisdictions still recognize *sovereign immunity*. The concept behind sovereign immunity is that the State can do no wrong. Because the State can do no wrong, such a policy, if practiced, applies only to public employees, and it applies only to claims of negligence that occurred in the performance of the employee's duties for the state. Most states have enacted laws removing sovereign immunity and now allow the State and its employees to be sued for negligence. Even in jurisdictions that still have sovereign immunity, sovereign immunity for public employees is a defense against negligence and not a bar to being sued. The employee will still have to pay to go to court and use the defense.

In an interesting trend associated with immunity laws, at least 12 states have enacted laws that provide immunity from ordinary negligence for volunteer coaches in youth sports programs.[7] As mentioned, under such laws coaches still have to pay to defend themselves, but the law does provide a total defense.

Such immunity is seen as an enticement to get more individuals into youth coaching. More and more coaches are needed because of the growth in youth sport, but apparently some do not volunteer for fear of being sued if anything happens. Provision of immunity as an enticement to these individuals sounds extremely negative in that it puts having a larger pool of coaches ahead of the safety of participants. This assumes that the right to sue if injuries occur is one way of assuring more diligence on the part of the coach to provide safe activities.

Some states that have enacted these laws have attempted to overcome this negative aspect by making the immunity applicable only to coaches who receive some low level of certification showing some level of competence in coaching. This is certainly a true transfer of liability for risks, but it would seem to be counter to good risk management.

Good Samaritan Laws

Good Samaritan laws

A final statute available in most states for the transference of liability are *Good Samaritan laws*. Whereas the statutes described above apply to situations in which the actor has a duty to the party who was injured, Good Samaritan laws apply to situations in which the actor had no duty to the injured party. These laws give immunity from ordinary negligence to persons who assist in accidents and are later sued by the accident victim. Without such laws, no one would stop to assist accident victims for fear of being sued. Good Samaritan laws can be general or specific. General laws typically apply to anyone who provides assistance. Specific laws apply only to certain persons, such as doctors or nurses. Professionals should be aware of the law in their jurisdiction.

Professionals should also be aware that Good Samaritan laws do not apply to persons who have a duty to act. Because this is true, it might seem that consideration of these laws is not a part of risk management or transfer of risks. During the course of their duties, however, exercise-related professionals may well experience situations in which they might need to assist persons to whom they have no duty. They might also be required to assist persons to whom they would not normally owe any duty but now do because of some special assignment. In either case, professionals should know whether they are an actor subject to the Good Samaritan laws. They will typically not know this unless it has been part of the information provided through a thorough risk analysis and risk management plan.

RECAP

In summary, the steps in risk management are:

1. Identify foreseeable risks.

2. Remove the risks that can be removed.

3. Control the risks that cannot be removed.

4. Transfer liability for risks when appropriate.

NOTES

1. L. J. Carpenter, *Legal Concepts in Sport: A Primer*. (Reston, VA: American Alliance for Health, Physical Education, Recreation and Dance, 1995).
2. Carpenter.
3. N. J. Dougherty, et al. *Sport, Physical Activity, and the Law*. (Champaign, IL: Human Kinetics, 1994).
4. Dougherty.
5. Dougherty.
6. Dougherty.
7. Carpenter.

RESOURCES

Appenzeller, H. (Ed.) (1985). *Sports and Law, Contemporary Issues*. Charlottesville, VA: Michie Co.

Appenzeller, H. (Ed.) (1998). *Risk Management in Sport, Issues and Strategies*. Durham, NC: Carolina Academic Press.

Hart, J. E., and R. J. Ritson. (1993). *Liability and Safety in Physical Education and Sport*. Reston, VA: American Alliance of Health, Physical Education, Recreation and Dance.

Nolan, J. R., and J. M. Nolan-Haley. (1990). *Black's Law Dictionary*, 6th ed. St. Paul: West Publishing.

Railey, J. H., and P. R. Tschauner. (1993). *Managing Physical Education, Fitness, and Sports Programs*. Mountain View, CA: Mayfield Publishing.

Van der Smissen, B. (1990–95). *Legal Liability and Risk Management for Public and Private Entities*. Cincinnati: Anderson Publishing.

Understanding Case Analysis

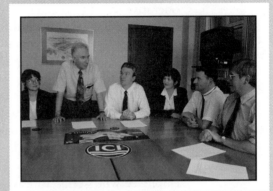

OBJECTIVES

After studying this chapter, you should be able to:

1. Identify and explain the steps of the case analysis process.

2. Utilize the case-analysis process to develop sound proposed solutions for a variety of administrative problems.

3. Identify and discuss the critical elements of a common administrative scenario.

4. Apply this same process to analyze and solve real-life administrative problems.

Effective decision-making is crucial to administrative success. As with critical skills of any type, sound decision-making strategies must be learned. They also must be practiced if they are to be mastered. One method of providing the student of administration with the opportunity to practice administrative decision-making in a non-threatening environment is known as *case analysis*. A hypothetical scenario (the case) is presented, and the student uses a systematic process to analyze the facts of the scenario and arrive at decisions designed to solve the problems arising from the scenario. As students become more comfortable with the analytic process, they will gain valuable decision-making expertise. As in real-world exercise-related administration, no one, single solution is applicable to all situations, with all other possibilities being unacceptable. Several solutions may be effective. Therefore, creative thinking is a valuable part of the case analysis process.

THE CASE ANALYSIS PROCESS

Several basic principles can enhance the ease and effectiveness of the case analysis process.

1. *Work independently, conducting your own analysis of the case.* Like most young professionals (teachers, coaches, athletic trainers, fitness specialists), the aspiring administrators frequently face the temptation of looking to others for assistance when problems arise. Even though this co-operative strategy is often encouraged in inexperienced professionals, the case analysis process should be undertaken independently rather than "cloning" the solution of a colleague.

2. *Master the facts of the case.* Each scenario contains numerous statements, opinions, inferences, and questions. The reader must identify all events that are present with sufficient credibility to be accepted as factual. For example, if the author of a case states that a principal character in the case (We will call her Mary) frequently criticizes or demeans employees publicly, the reader may conclude that this behavior is factual. If, however, the statement about Mary's behavior comes from a fellow employee who seems to have a personality conflict with Mary, one may question the credibility of the statement and, therefore, consider it an opinion rather than a fact. This decision should be made carefully, as it may impact the identification of a specific problem to be solved and the ultimate proposed solution.

The reader may find it helpful to highlight or underline each fact in preparation for listing the facts on the case analysis form. Once all facts have been identified, the next step is to separate the facts that are essential to the problem from those that are extraneous. This will enable one to focus on relevant issues.

3. *Identify the principal characters in the case.* Throughout the fact-identification step, the reader should make note of all the characters in the case. As with the facts, highlighting or underlining in a different color may make the task easier. Then the reader should carefully consider the extent to which each character is pertinent to the problem presented and/or the potential solution. People who seem to have no real impact on the problem or its potential solution should be eliminated. Those remaining are considered principal characters.

4. *Recognize biases and prejudices in the case.* Careful analysis may reveal what seems to be bias or prejudice on the part of one or more of the characters. Bias or prejudice should be taken into consideration when evaluating the substance of the character's statements or actions. Suspected bias or prejudice should be supported by evidence (past actions, statements, and so forth) rather than merely a hunch.

5. *Identify the specific problem before attempting to propose a solution.* Have you ever shared a problem with friends only to have them begin to offer advice before they fully understand the problem? That approach is similar to a baseball player who runs around the bases before hitting the ball. It may be enjoyable, but it accomplishes nothing. The case must be studied carefully to determine the specific problems before attempting to arrive at the appropriate solution.

6. *Base proposed solutions on sound administrative reasoning.* Proposing solutions based upon personal opinion is easy to do. A person with no administrative education, expertise, or experience can offer solutions. One of the main purposes of the case-analysis process is to make decisions based on sound administrative reasoning rather than on personal opinion. Therefore, all solutions should be accompanied by written justification, including specific administrative principles, concepts, and reasoning upon which the proposed solution is based.

Relevant principles and concepts can be found not only in this book, but also in many other professional resources. Although the Internet has become a popular source of information, one should be cautious when using Internet information. Because the Internet is largely unregulated, information found there is not necessarily from a reputable source and, therefore, should be used only if taken from a written source for which documentation is available.

THE CASE ANALYSIS REPORT

The case analysis should be presented in the form of a written report. A simple case analysis report form is presented in Figure 17.1.

Brief Overview of the Case

This section should contain no more than two or three sentences giving a thumbnail sketch of the case. Example: "This case involves a secondary school physical education teacher who also serves as assistant girls basketball coach. Her teaching duties and coaching responsibilities have begun to create a time conflict during the last teaching period of the day (just prior to the beginning of basketball practice). She would like to give up her coaching role but has been told that if she does not coach, she will be transferred to an elementary school, and she does not feel qualified to teach elementary physical education."

Principal Characters

Principal characters are listed, along with brief descriptive information about each. This descriptive information may include things such as the character's job title, former position, and relationship to one or more of the other characters. Example: "The principal characters in this case are:

1. Dr. Richards, President of I.Q. University
2. Mr. Williams, Athletics Director at I.Q. University
3. Mrs. Abbot, President of I.Q. Athletic Booster Club
4. Coach Crawford, Assistant Athletics Director for Men's Sports
5. Ms. Stockwell, Assistant Athletics Director for Women's Sports"

Essential Facts

This part of the report tends to be the most lengthy, as many facts are usually considered essential to the case. Facts should be stated concisely, yet accurately. If biases or prejudices are present in evaluating the facts, these should be clearly stated, along with evidence of bias or prejudice. Example: "The essential facts in this case are:

1. The university has two certified athletic trainers.
2. Both athletic trainers (head trainer and assistant trainer) are male.
3. The university has 10 sports teams — 5 men's teams and 5 women's teams.
4. The university is conducting a self-study in preparation for implementing a new degree program in athletic training.

Case Analysis Report Form

I.   Brief Overview:

II.   Principal Characters:

III. Essential Facts:

FIGURE 17.1

IV.   Specific Major Problems:

V.   Specific Sub-Problems (if any):

VI.   Proposed Solution(s):
           Immediate/Current

           Long-Term

VII.   Justification:
           Immediate/Current

           Long-Term

FIGURE 17.1 *Continued*

5. The university's president and chief academic officer disagree about the need for hiring a third athletic trainer.

6. Etc."

Specific Major Problems

This is likely to be the most difficult part of the process. What appears to be the obvious problem may not be. A more careful analysis may indicate several problems, many or all of which may not be immediately obvious. Each specific problem should be listed and briefly described.

The specific problems in this case are:

1. An unresolved personality conflict between Jim Andrus and Suzie Ketner, fitness instructors in Mercy Hospital's HealthFit Program.

2. Mercy Hospital's HealthFit Program is under the direction of the hospital's Director of Nursing, whose office is in the hospital, not at the HealthFit facility, across town from the hospital.

Specific Sub-Problems (If Any)

Major problems are often the direct result of existing smaller problems. Therefore, the solution to the major problem may lie in solving the sub-problems that are causing it. When sub-problems are identified, they should be listed and briefly described. This case has two specific sub-problems:

1. The cardiac rehabilitation program cannot offer first aid/CPR courses for the family members of program participants without having a certified instructor.

2. The new cardiac rehabilitation assistant cannot obtain her instructor's certification until she receives her basic first aid/CPR certification.

Proposed Solutions

Solutions to most administrative problems must be proposed and enacted at two levels. An *immediate* or *current solution* must be found to alleviate the problem in the present. A *long-term solution* must be enacted to prevent (hopefully eliminate) recurrence of the problem in the future. These proposed solutions should be stated specifically and tied directly to the specific problems for which they are proposed. Example: "For Problem #1 (the Assistant Director of Events Planning's repeated failure to submit monthly budget reports on time), proposed solutions are:

Immediate/Current

Assign one of the existing sport management interns to the Assistant Director to collect, maintain, and enter budget data into the computer throughout the month. This will reduce the Assistant Director's heavy workload — the apparent reason for his problem with getting budget reports in on time. This should solve the immediate problem.

Long-Term

Review the Assistant Director's position description and determine what specific responsibilities can be realistically shifted to another staff member, thereby providing the Assistant Director with a more reasonable workload. For example, taking away the supervisory responsibility for sport management interns from the Assistant Director and giving it to the specific department heads within which the interns work will allow the Assistant Director more time to collect budget data and prepare budget reports. This should provide a long-term solution for the problem.

Justification

The final step in the case analysis report is the statement of justification containing the specific administrative principles, concepts, or reasoning (along with appropriate documentation) upon which each proposed solution is based.

Each principle, concept, or statement of rationale must be tied directly to the specific proposed solution for which it is being used as justification. For Problem #1 (the Assistant Director of Events Planning's repeated failure to submit monthly budget reports on time), the justification for each proposed solution is as follows:

Immediate/Current

The results of a personnel performance analysis indicated that the Assistant Director's poor performance was related to an E/C (Environmental/Circumstantial) problem (excessive workload, which prevented him from meeting his budget report deadlines). Therefore, the appropriate solution must be administrative intervention to remove the E/C problem [see Chapter 9].

Long-Term

A review of the span of control and position responsibilities of each member of the organization revealed that the responsibilities of the Assistant Director for Events Planning had been expanded, creating the E/C problem cited above. When an employee's span of control is too broad, one appropriate solution is to reduce the employee's span of control by modifying the existing organizational structure [see Chapter 3].

DISCUSSION OF CASE ANALYSIS

An essential part of the case analysis learning process is the open discussion of cases, their analysis, and the proposed solutions. Discussion presents an opportunity to share perspectives and analytic reasoning while learning from peers. In a class situation, the instructor's role should be that of an impartial discussion facilitator, waiting until the conclusion of the discussion to offer their perspective. This allows the instructor the opportunity to share alternative solutions the students did not offer, without becoming the central figure in the discussion/sharing/learning time. A few suggestions will enhance the effectiveness of the discussion.

1. *Listen carefully to everything that is said.* One of the most effective ways to gain a broader knowledge is by listening (taking notes also helps) to the perspectives of everyone engaged in the discussion. Some will offer comments that agree with your analysis, and others will hold an opposing position. The goal here is learning, and much can be learned from listening to others' ideas.

2. *Weigh the ideas presented by others before accepting or rejecting them.* Listen to the comments with an open mind. An idea that sounds great on the surface may lack appropriate depth or justification, whereas an idea that seems to be off base may actually open your mind to a host of creative ideas. Accepting or rejecting the ideas of others before considering their merits deprives you of the opportunity to think creatively.

3. *Don't propose solutions simply to gain approval of peers or the instructor or to entertain classmates.* Proposed solutions should be based upon a careful and thorough analysis of the facts of the case and sound administrative justification. Proposing a solution for the purpose of gaining approval or to liven up the discussion would deprive you of the opportunity to think independently and creatively and deprive others of the opportunity to learn from your comments and ideas.

RESOURCES

Zeigler, E. F. (1982). *Decision-Making in Physical Education and Athletics Administration: A Case Method Approach.* Champaign, IL: Stipes Publishing.

Case Analysis Activities: Physical Education and Athletics

18

Case Scenario 18A

Briarcliff Academy — Who's in Charge

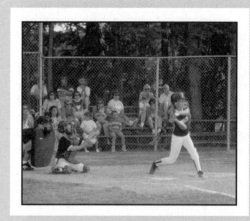

Briarcliff Academy is a private school with an enrollment of 450 students in grades 1–12. The school had just completed its first year of operation, during which the school's athletics program consisted of high school and junior high school basketball and high school baseball. Being their first year of competition, the Cliff Dwellers athletics teams won few games but enjoyed tremendous support from fans. The fact that the school had no athletics facilities did not dampen school spirit.

Briarcliff is governed by a board of directors composed of local doctors, attorneys, farmers, businessmen, and businesswomen. Mr. Ross, chairman of the board, is owner of

a local insurance agency and has had no prior experience in educational administration. Speaking for the board on several occasions, he stated that the academy's first priority is a strong, science-oriented academic program. He often speaks of the value of athletics and of the board's desire to see a successful basketball program at Briarcliff. Although the board has no plans to expand the athletics program at the present time, the community clearly would like to see the academy start a football program.

At the conclusion of the academy's inaugural year, Coach Glen, the school's basketball and baseball coach and physical education instructor, resigned because of what he called his "unfair workload" (3 physical education classes, 3 science classes, and coaching responsibilities for both basketball and baseball).

Mr. Lynn, Briarcliff's principal, began his search for Coach Glen's replacement and, in the meantime, was advised by the board of directors that the school would start a football program the following year. This, it was decided, made it necessary to hire two teachers/coaches — one for football and one for basketball and baseball. Mr. Lynn, a former basketball coach, decided to coach the junior high basketball team, leaving the new basketball coach with responsibility for only the high school team.

As a result of Mr. Lynn's search, Coach Dale was invited to the school to interview for the football coaching position. Coach Dale had just completed his master's degree work in physical education and had both playing and coaching experience in football, basketball, track, and tennis. The board of director decided that Dale's experience and background in science and music made him the best person for the coaching position.

Coach Dale accepted the job of starting the academy's junior high school football program, with the understanding that when the program would expand to the high school level, he would have the option of coaching the varsity team or remaining as the coach of the junior high team. He agreed to teach three physical education classes and two music classes in addition to coaching football.

Prior to the beginning of the school year, Mr. Lynn asked Coach Dale if he would consider teaching one science class, as he had earned a minor in biology in college, and the projected increase in enrollment made an additional science class necessary. Coach Dale reluctantly agreed to the arrangement but only after being assured that every attempt would be made to eliminate the science class the following year.

As the start of school approached, Mr. Lynn was unsuccessful in finding a suitable candidate for the varsity basketball coaching vacancy. Therefore, Coach Dale was asked to serve as basketball coach for one year and was given an additional stipend.

The school year went smoothly, with both the football and basketball teams winning championships. Coach Dale was extremely busy with his many duties, but the support of the local fans and success of the football and basketball programs seemed to make all the extra work worthwhile.

During football season Coach Dale was assisted by Mr. Camp, the school's math teacher, who had no athletics experience but was willing to learn, and Mr. Weldon, the school's chemistry and physics teacher and baseball coach, who had played high school football and earned a minor in physical education in college. Coach Dale's and Mr. Weldon's coaching philosophies were quite different, resulting in several disagreements, though none of major proportions. Mr. Lynn often suggested to Coach Dale that he "go along with Mr. Weldon's methods" to "keep peace," so Coach Dale usually used a combination of both philosophies to appease Mr. Lynn.

When spring rolled around, contracts for the upcoming year were issued to the teachers for their consideration. When Coach Dale received his contract, he was shocked to find that it called for him to teach six classes and coach basketball instead of football. Coach Dale immediately contacted Mr. Lynn, who said that contract details were determined by the board of directors. Coach Dale then telephoned Mr. Ross to ask why the contract stipulated basketball instead of football. Mr. Ross told him that the board was so pleased with the success of the basketball team that it decided Coach Dale was the best person to continue as basketball coach. Mr. Ross also stated that, because Mr. Weldon had football playing experience, assigning him the football coaching duties would reduce Coach Dale's load. When Coach Dale attempted to protest, Mr. Ross informed him that Mr. Weldon had already returned his signed contract, so nothing further could be done. The next day, Coach Dale overheard Mr. Weldon telling a colleague that his new contract required him to teach only five classes, which made Coach Dale even angrier.

After several conversations between Coach Dale and members of the board of directors, Dale agreed to return as basketball coach if the promise to reduce his teaching load to five classes could be worked out. After considering the request, the board announced that the six-class load should not be reduced because (1) physical education requires little or no planning time and (2) taking away his football coaching duties had already reduced his load.

During the ensuing weeks, Coach Dale received many requests from parents, students, and fellow teachers to accept the contract as offered. While pondering his decision, Coach Dale inadvertently ran into a sporting goods salesman who called on Briarcliff during the school year and was told that Mr. Lynn had informed him during basketball season that Mr. Weldon would be the new football coach at Briarcliff. Coach Dale simply did not know what to do.

Case Analysis Report Form
18A – Briarcliff Academy — Who's in charge?

I. Brief Overview:

II. Principal Characters:

III. Essential Facts:

IV. Specific Major Problems:

V. Specific Sub-problems (if any):

VI. Proposed Solutions:

    Immediate/Current

    Long-Term

VII. Justification:

Case Scenario 18B

Jessup College — Who's Number 1

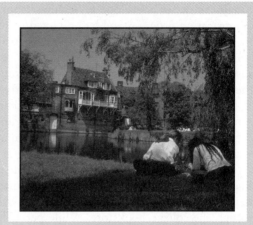

Jessup College is a small northeastern liberal arts college with an enrollment of 1,500 students. For the past 2 years, Dr. Temple has been employed as a temporary full-time faculty member at Jessup. His specific position is Coordinator of Sport Administration for the undergraduate major program in sport administration. His teaching assignments have included courses in sport marketing, sport law, and event management. Dr. Temple, or "Dr. T," as the students fondly call him, is highly popular with the Jessup students. Many students consider him as much a friend as a professor. Students characterize his classes as "engaging" and "fun."

This past spring, the Coordinator of Sport Administration was converted to a tenure track position. Dr. Temple was clearly a front-runner for the position, but, according to college policy, the college was required to conduct a national search for the position. The search committee was headed by Dr. Clark, chair of the Department of Exercise & Sport Science (EES). The remaining EES faculty made up the search committee.

Applications poured in from around the country, representing many fine candidates for

the position. After carefully reading the letters of application, vitae, and letters of recommendation, phone calls were placed to selected references to check on credentials. Based upon all the information gathered, the search committee identified three finalists for the position — Dr. Temple and two external candidates.

A series of on-campus interviews was arranged for each candidate with a variety of college administrators and faculty members and staff members. Each candidate was also required to teach a "sample class" on a topic of choice related to sport marketing, sport law, or event management. Following each candidate's campus visit, feedback was gathered from as many sources as possible.

The first candidate to visit the Jessup campus was Dr. Stevens, a professor from a major midwestern university. Her visit was followed by that of Dr. Mawsen, a department chair from a small southern college. Dr. Temple was the last candidate to complete the interview/teaching process.

On the surface, everything seemed to be going smoothly. Everyone openly acknowledged that the process had to be somewhat awkward for Dr. Temple, as he had played a major role in developing Jessup's sport administration program and had directed it for the past 2 years. Likewise, the process was somewhat uncomfortable for the students because they felt an allegiance to "Dr. T." Yet another source of awkwardness stemmed from the fact that Dr. Temple and Dr. Mawsen had been faculty colleagues for several years at another institution prior to Dr. Temple's arrival at Jessup.

During Dr. Mawsen's campus visit, something unexpected happened. Between scheduled interviews, Dr. Mawsen decided to browse through the college bookstore. While perusing the sport administration section, he noticed that the required text for one of Dr. Temple's courses was a bound collection of handouts and article reprints. As Dr. Mawsen thumbed through the collection, he immediately recognized a number of materials as his own. Yet, there they were in their original form, but with Dr. Temple's name on them.

At dinner that evening, Dr. Mawsen told Dr. Clark about his discovery. Dr. Clark's heart sank. Was the information true? If so, this was an obvious case of plagiarism — a most serious affront to academic integrity. Dr. Clark asked Dr. Mawsen if he could send her original copies of the materials from his file as "evidence" of his claim. Dr. Mawsen agreed to provide original drafts of the material as soon as he returned to his campus. In the meantime, Dr. Clark told no one else of the incident.

As expected, Dr. Temple's interviews and sample teaching went well. Based upon the interviews, sample lessons, and feedback from administrators, faculty, staff, and students, the search committee's decision had all indications of being an easy one. While all three candidates were well qualified, were well received by the campus community, and appeared to be a "good fit" for the position, Dr. Temple's experience and performance at Jessup made him the clear choice for the position. Dr. Mawsen was ranked number 2, and Dr. Stevens was ranked number 3.

Dr. Clark soon received the promised materials from Dr. Mawsen. Her fears seemed to be confirmed. In her opinion, Dr. Temple was guilty of blatant plagiarism. Dr. Clark called an emergency meeting of the search committee and shared the information. Following the meeting, she also advised the college President and Academic Dean.

What should they do? Was this apparent plagiarism a "red flag" sufficient to eliminate Dr. Temple from consideration for the position? If not, could Dr. Clark and the other faculty members work with a colleague who had violated such an essential principle of academia? If Dr. Temple is not offered the position, then who? If Dr. Mawsen is hired, could there be further "fallout?" Maybe Dr. Stevens should be hired, as both Dr. Temple and Dr. Mawsen were involved in the incident. And what should the students be told?

Case Analysis Report Form
18B – Jessup College — Who's Number 1?

I. Brief Overview:

II. Principal Characters:

III. Essential Facts:

IV. Specific Major Problems:

V. Specific Sub-problems (if any):

VI. Proposed Solutions:

Immediate/Current

Long-Term

VII. Justification:

Case Scenario 18C

Larkin High School — Come on . . . Dunk One!

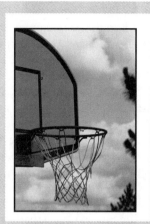

Larkin High School is a typical small-town high school with an enrollment of 500 students in grades 9–12. Ninth grade students who as eighth graders had performed poorly on state-mandated standardized tests were required to take part in a math enrichment class. Each class consists of 10 students, taught by a classroom teacher during the seventh (last) period of the school day. Students generally have a rather low opinion of the math enrichment classes and often state that they do not understand why these are required of certain students. The goal of the requirement, however, is to prepare the students for the standardized tests they must pass so they can graduate.

In an attempt to motivate students participating in the class, teachers are encouraged to develop and use positive reinforcement strategies when possible. Some of the common rewards approved by the school principal have been snacks, movies, and special games. Students may earn these rewards by successfully completing units in the enrichment course.

Chris McGuire, a math teacher at the school, was one of the math enrichment instructors. Mr. McGuire thought his students

would enjoy free-play time in the school gymnasium and asked the principal if that would be an acceptable reward. McGuire also believed this would offer an excellent opportunity for him to develop teacher-student camaraderie by joining the students in their play. Because the gym was not used for physical education classes during seventh period, the principal approved Mr. McGuire's request.

Mr. McGuire arranged to have the gym lights left on, and borrowed basketballs from the physical education teachers. For security purposes, all coaches' offices, locker rooms, and storage rooms were locked prior to seventh period. Mr. McGuire was anxious to see how his students would respond to his new reward.

At the conclusion of the first math enrichment unit, Mr. McGuire was thrilled by the performance of his students. Apparently the promise of free-play time in the gym had been just the motivator he had been looking for. On Friday afternoon, Mr. McGuire's seventh-period math enrichment class met in the gym. Although all the students had physical education clothes in their gym lockers, they were unable to change into them because the locker rooms were locked. Teams were chosen from among the students who wanted to play basketball, with the remaining students allowed to sit in the bleachers and talk, draw, or do homework. Mr. McGuire played basketball with the "more serious" players.

As time went by, Mr. McGuire's reward system became so popular among the students that other math enrichment classes asked their teachers to let them have gym time. The other teachers, however, did not share Mr. McGuire's enthusiasm for the idea. Personally, Mr. McGuire was happy that none of the other classes came to the gym, as he thought it made his students feel special and enhanced the motivational effect. Besides, he was thrilled with the opportunity to get a good workout himself.

On Friday afternoon, following the successful completion of another math enrichment unit, the class headed off for its much-anticipated gym time. Jason Smith, a rather nonathletic student, took his usual place in the bleachers to watch the other students play basketball.

Because he is 6'5" tall, when people see Jason, they often assume he is a basketball player. While sitting in the bleachers, one of the other students began to tease Jason, betting him that he could not dunk a basketball. Jason left the bleachers and effortlessly dunked a basketball at an unattended basket. Even Jason himself was surprised at the ease with which he was able to dunk the ball.

After several successful dunks, Jason misjudged his jump and fell hard to the floor. He cried out in pain, obviously hurt seriously. When Mr. McGuire got to Jason, he saw that the fractured bone in Jason's upper arm had broken through the skin. Jason was rushed to the hospital, where he underwent several hours of emergency surgery. The following morning Jason's father telephoned the principal to say, "My wife and I are on our way to your office. We have a lot of questions about what happened to Jason, and you had better have some answers!"

Case Analysis Report Form
18C – Larkin High School — Come on . . . Dunk One!

I. Brief Overview:

II. Principal Characters:

III. Essential Facts:

IV. Specific Major Problems:

V. Specific Sub-problems (if any):

VI. Proposed Solutions:

Immediate/Current

Long-Term

VII. Justification:

Case Scenario 18D

Dodge College — Budget, Budget, Who Has the Budget?

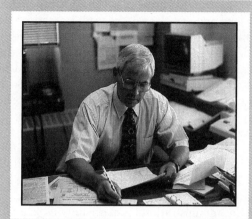

Harvey Hogan was in his 31st year as Athletics Director at Dodge College, a coeducational, private liberal arts college that offered 13 sports and was a member of the strong Champions Intercollegiate Athletic Conference (CIAC). Hogan was proud of the fact that, although his athletics budget was the smallest in the 10-school conference, he had always operated in the black. A serious enrollment problem had developed over the past two years, however, and the number of students enrolled at Dodge College had dropped dramatically. As a result of the enrollment crisis, each department was cautioned that it would go to a B budget if the enrollment did not increase significantly for the upcoming year. Ms. Newman, the college's chief financial officer (CFO) told all department heads that their individual budgets could not go over the designated amount.

Hogan met with his coaches and apprised them of the financial crisis that faced the college. He asked for their help but really did not foresee a problem because the Athletics Department had never gone over budget in his 30 years as Athletics Director.

The fiscal year ended on June 1, and Hogan received an emergency call from Ms.

Newman on June 15, asking him to meet the following day to explain why he was over budget by $12,000. She told him that four sports had exceeded their allotted budgets and reported that men's basketball, women's volleyball, men's tennis, and football were the violators. Ms. Newman was obviously distraught and highly agitated. Hogan immediately called each coach who had exceeded the budget to explain how they had failed to comply with his request to "hold the line."

The women's volleyball coach had failed to check her monthly computer printouts because she was "too busy coaching and recruiting" to spend time on the printout. She said she was sure she was within budget. Upon investigation, the coach admitted that she was thrilled to be asked to chaperone the intramural flag football team to the national tournament in New Orleans and had transferred funds to the intramural team's budget to help fund the trip to New Orleans. In addition, she paid for their uniforms from her volleyball budget. She regretted the overage and stated that it was the first time this had ever happened.

The football coach could not believe that he had gone over his budget by $5,000. Upon investigation he found that the dry cleaner that washed and dry-cleaned the team's practice and game equipment had failed to send a monthly bill as requested. Instead, the owner of the cleaning establishment waited until the end of school to send a $5,000 bill. The football coach was devastated because his budget was the largest in the department and a source of criticism by students and faculty who wanted the sport dropped because they thought it was too costly for a small college. He had been sensitive to the criticism and had tried to stay within his budget. He also had been under heavy criticism by the administration for exceeding his scholarship limit.

In previous years, several students who were offered grants-in-aid did not report for practice, choosing to enroll at other schools. He was certain this would happen again, but fortunately or unfortunately, every scholarship athlete reported for practice, and he was over by two grants ($40,000). Though he was still in compliance with CIAC rules, he was over the institution's limit.

The men's tennis coach had always ignored Ms. Newman's directive to turn in all receipts by June 1. Instead he regularly procrastinated until as late as mid-July, when he would turn in receipts for the national tournament held in May. He was $2,000 over budget.

Men's lacrosse exceeded its budget because the coach, who had built a nationally ranked team, had decided during the season to take a northern road trip to play several games during spring break. He had no excuse other than that he thought the road trip against tough competition would help his national ranking and be good publicity for the college and help his recruiting.

In addition to the critical overage, another serious problem surfaced. The track-and-field coach had asked for his own personal computer. After he was told that his request could not be approved this year but would be considered for the following year, he worked a deal with a local computer store. The salesperson agreed to let him get a computer and hold the bill until the following year, when he was told he could purchase a computer.

Unfortunately, the computer salesperson was fired. The owner of the computer company found out about the bill and called Ms. Newman, demanding payment. A final item of frustration was when Mr. Hogan received a bill without a proper code to identify which sport had ordered 12 dozen pairs of athletic socks. No one admitted to having ordered the socks, and it was a mystery as to how the purchase order got through the business office without approval of the Athletics Director, who was required to sign all purchase orders.

Ms. Newman was furious and phoned Mr. Hogan to ask, "Who is in control of the Athletics Department budget — you or your coaches?"

Case Analysis Report Form
18D – Dodge College — Budget, Budget, Who Has the Budget?

I. Brief Overview:

II. Principal Characters:

III. Essential Facts:

IV. Specific Major Problems:

V. Specific Sub-problems (if any):

VI. Proposed Solutions:

Immediate/Current

Long-Term

VII. Justification:

Case Scenario 18E

Hartsfield University — Celebration Turns Ugly

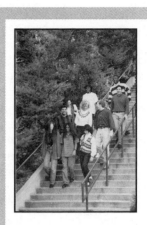

Hartsfield University is a small liberal arts university located in a midwestern city of 50,000. The Hartsfield student population represents every state, and even several foreign countries. The student body includes individuals of all races, ethnicities, socioeconomic classes, and sexual orientations. The student body is intentionally diverse because Hartsfield prides itself on recognizing the value of all human beings. The college has had an official nondiscrimination policy for more than 20 years. The university's nondiscrimination statement purports that the university does not discriminate in admissions or educational programming. Specifically identified in the nondiscrimination statement are race, religion, ethnicity, sexual orientation, marital status, and physical abilities. Educational content related to social justice has a prominent place in the curriculum at Hartsfield, and a number of student organizations work to promote understanding of diversity and to further the cause of social justice.

For the past several years, the Gay, Lesbian, Bisexual, and Allies Student Association (GLBASA) has celebrated October as Gay History Month. Throughout the month, the

GLBASA members host a series of educational and social events to raise awareness and to educate the college community about the concerns of gays, lesbians, and bisexuals. As has been the tradition, this past October began with early-morning decorating of the lobby of the Student Union building by GLBASA members. Students entering the Union could not miss the rainbow flags, banners, and posters announcing Gay History Month. On the sidewalks leading to the Union were colorful chalk drawings (approved by the administration) with slogans such as, "Love knows no gender" and "Hate is not a family value."

Many students (gay, bisexual, and straight) and faculty looked forward to a poetry reading scheduled for October 1 at 9 pm. The event would be the first official Gay History Month activity. Attendance at the poetry reading was good, and those who attended left feeling proud about the level of acceptance (or at least tolerance) in the university community. As attendees at the poetry reading exited through the lobby, however, they were shocked by what they saw. While the poetry reading was in progress, someone (or someones) had ripped down the banners and defaced the posters and rainbow flags. On the sidewalks outside, the chalk drawings had been replaced with alternative messages such as, "Burn the faggots" and "Gay = Sick." People wondered who would do such a thing.

By the next day, the answer was apparent. The perpetrators had been observed doing their damage by two students who accidentally came upon them while passing through to get snacks from the snack room. These students, Jane and Sue, just happened to be writers for *The Hartsfield Voice*, the university newspaper. Jane and Sue met separately with Dr. Jefferson, the Dean of Students. Their accounts of the events were similar as they told Dr. Jefferson that there were five or possibly six perpetrators. Although neither Jane nor Sue knew any of the men by name, they both said they recognized all or at least some of them as members of the university's football team.

Upon hearing this, Dr. Jefferson immediately called Mr. Kline, the university's Director of Athletics. In turn, Mr. Kline called Coach Long, the head football coach, into his office, and told him to "get to the bottom of this — now." Mr. Kline recognized that this incident had the potential for a lot of negative publicity for the Athletics Department if not handled properly.

That afternoon, Coach Long canceled practice and met with the team in a large lecture hall on campus. He told the players about the charges being leveled. He admitted to them that "I don't like fags any more than anyone else" but insisted that tolerance was expected behavior for all Hartsfield athletes. He then went around the room and asked each player if he knew anything about the incident. One by one, each football player denied any knowledge of the incident.

Coach Long returned to his office, where he immediately placed a voice-mail message to both Dr. Jefferson and Mr. Kline. His message stated that he was "positive" that none of his players was involved in the incident, so the students who reported the information must either be mistaken or lying. Coach Long assumed that this was the end of the issue.

The next morning, an editorial in *The Hartsfield Voice* announced that members of the school's football team had been seen defacing the Gay History Month decorations. The editorial suggested that the Athletics Department has a responsibility to identify and punish the guilty players and to educate *all* of the university's student athletes about the "dangers of homophobia."

Case Analysis Report Form
18E – Hartsfield University . . . Celebration Turns Ugly

I. Brief Overview:

II. Principal Characters:

III. Essential Facts:

IV. Specific Major Problems:

V. Specific Sub-problems (if any):

VI. Proposed Solutions:

Immediate/Current

Long-Term

VII. Justification:

Case Scenario 18F

Denmark High School — Something Rotten in Denmark

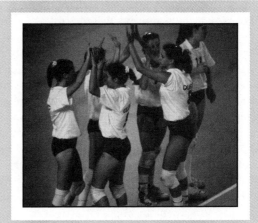

Christine was thrilled with her new position as physical education instructor and girl's volleyball coach at Denmark High School. During her first semester on the job, she spent a significant amount of time preparing for her classes because she was committed to quality physical education instruction, and many of her students tended to view physical education as free-play time. She also devoted a lot of time to developing a successful volleyball program, as Denmark had never been very competitive in the sport. Although DHS had had a volleyball team for 6 years, it had never had a winning season. With her dedication to quality teaching and coaching, Christine had little time left for herself.

Before long, Christine began to reap the rewards of her commitment. At the end of her first semester, students openly praised her as "the best physical education teacher we've ever had." Not only was her volleyball team winning, but their cumulative gradepoint average for the first semester was 3.2. Ms. McDonald, Head of the Physical Education Department, was extremely pleased with Christine, having

been instrumental in her hiring. Her colleagues recognized Christine's commitment to developing quality *student* athletes and were quick to include her in both school and social activities.

In Christine's mind, she and Denmark High School were "a match made in heaven." Little did she know that something was rotten at Denmark. The more successful her volleyball team became, the more she experienced difficulties with the school's Athletics Director and Head Basketball Coach, Mr. Kavolchick (or Coach K, as the the students called him).

Despite the fact that the volleyball team was in second place in its conference, it was constantly the butt of jokes in Coach K's science classes. In fact, some of the players were in Coach K's class when, after its first match, he joked, "Well, the volleyball team is undefeated (at 1–0) for the first, and probably last, time in school history." Everyone laughed heartily — everyone, that is, except the volleyball players. To make matters worse, the players told Christine that Coach K was constantly saying, "Okay, girls, pay close attention, now. You know these science problems are more difficult for you females." Christine tried to ignore Coach K's comments and reassured her players that the comments were harmless.

When Christine made simple requests for her volleyball program, she was most often turned down. For example, when she asked Coach K if her volleyball girls could plan some fundraising events, she was told that those events might interfere with the football team's fundraising projects. The only way he would approve fundraising events for the volleyball team was if Christine would agree to give half of the money raised to the football program. Christine asked permission to host a large volleyball tournament in hopes of attracting area college coaches, but the request was denied, despite the fact that the boy's soccer program had hosted just such an event each year.

When Christine requested detailed information regarding her budget, she was given inaccurate figures. When she tried to reserve the Athletic Department van for an "away" match, she was told that it was scheduled to be in the shop for an oil change that day. When she met with Coach K to discuss her concerns, he became angry. As she turned to walk out of his office, he grabbed her by the jacket and said, "This meeting isn't over 'til *I* say it's over!"

Meanwhile, Christine was becoming aware of other problems in the school's athletics program. Coach Swikert, the Head Football Coach, repeatedly asked her to change the grades of some his players in her physical education class. This, he argued, would not only allow them to remain eligible but also would certainly help them earn college scholarships. From his perspective, Christine would be "providing a helping hand to students in need." When she steadfastly refused, some of her volleyball players began to complain of ill treatment in Coach Swikert's classes.

It was also common knowledge around the Athletics Department that some coaches arranged opportunities for college coaches to observe and talk with athletes more frequently than state high school league rules allowed. Athletes in classes taught by coaches routinely received A's, despite numerous absences and poor academic performance. The final straw was when Christine discovered that Coach K commonly shifted funds from the budgets of female sports into the football and boys' basketball budgets to cover overspending by those sports ("After all, football and boy's basketball bring in most of the money").

Christine was perplexed. Something was rotten in Denmark, all right!

Case Analysis Report Form
18F – Denmark High School — Something Rotten at Denmark!

I. Brief Overview:

II. Principal Characters:

III. Essential Facts:

IV. Specific Major Problems:

V. Specific Sub-problems (if any):

VI. Proposed Solutions:

Immediate/Current

Long-Term

VII. Justification:

Case Analysis Activities: Athletic Training and Sports Medicine

19

Case Scenario 19A

South Hills High School — But You Can't Get There from Here!

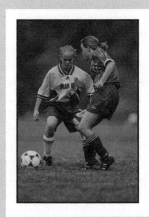

S outh Hills High School is located in a fast-growing northeast suburban community. In the past 5 years the school has experienced a tremendous increase in student enrollment. In response to the growing student body, Mr. Marks, South Hills' Athletics Director, proposed to the Board of Education that girls' varsity soccer, girls' junior varsity soccer, and junior varsity football be added to the existing sports program. In accordance with the school district's interscholastic athletics schedule, the three new teams would compete during the fall sports season.

One of the first people with whom Mr. Marks shared the good news of the Board's approval of the new sports was Julie O'Neil. Julie is an NATA-certified athletic trainer who was hired 2 years ago to provide medical coverage for South Hills' sports teams. Having played Division I football, Mr. Marks understood the importance of good medical care and the benefits of having a full-time NATA-certified athletic trainer. He had invested a great deal of time and effort to obtain funding for the Athletic Trainer position and frequently speaks of his belief that every practice and competition involving South Hills students should have an athletic trainer in attendance.

When Julie first arrived at South Hills, she was given a modest budget for ordering athletic training supplies. A storage room located adjacent to the boys' locker room was converted into a small, but functional athletic training room. Not wanting to spend the entire first-year budget on equipping the athletic training room, Julie acquired donated wood and built taping tables, shelves for storing coolers and supplies, and even a small table where she could do daily record-keeping.

Shortly after the fall sports season began, students began to contact Julie expressing interest in learning more about athletic training while gaining hands-on experience helping Julie. Having served as a student athletic trainer in high school herself, Julie eagerly worked to develop an effective student athletic training program.

Upon hearing the news of the three new sports teams, Julie was excited for the students who now would have the opportunity to participate in interscholastic sports. She also had a sense of panic at the thought of providing athletic training services for the new athletes during a fall season that was already a hectic time of the sports year. After considerable thought, she was comforted by the knowledge that the school had only two athletic fields, which traditionally had been used by the varsity football and boys' soccer teams. She drew the logical conclusion that the three new teams would practice on the two existing fields so it would

just mean longer practice days for her and her student athletic trainers.

Two weeks prior to the opening of school, Julie received a memo from Mr. Marks in which he enthusiastically explained how, through his hard work, the school had struck a deal with the city's Parks and Recreation Department to lease three of its athletic fields for the fall. The memo detailed the location of these practice fields and stated that they would be used exclusively by the three new teams. According to Mr. Marks' description, the leased fields could be reached by walking approximately one-quarter of a mile through a wooded area behind the school.

Following Mr. Marks' directions, Julie walked from the school to the leased practice fields, and what she found disturbed her. Although well-maintained, the fields were a significant distance from the nearest road, and, with the wooded area between the school and fields, they were inaccessible by car. In addition, there was no telephone in sight. Julie's professional preparation and experience had taught her that, in the event of a life-threatening medical emergency, it would be virtually impossible to get proper medical assistance to the new fields. So Julie wrote a detailed memo to Mr. Marks explaining her concerns.

The next day, Julie found the following memo in her school mailbox:

TO: Julie O'Neil, ATC
FROM: William Marks, Athletics Director
RE: Newly leased practice fields

After much thoughtful consideration of your concerns about the location of the newly acquired practice fields, I have decided to proceed with our agreement with the Parks and Recreation Department. I have, however, decided that the new fields will be used by the boys' varsity soccer team, the girls' varsity soccer team, and the boys' junior varsity soccer team. The football teams will practice on the school's practice fields, which are located adjacent to the school building. I understand your concern for the health and safety of the student-athletes. However, there are no other available practice facilities, and the opening of school is less than 2 weeks away. I'm sure everything will work out just fine.

Case Analysis Report Form
19A – South Hills High School — But You Can't Get There from Here!

I. Brief Overview:

II. Principal Characters:

III. Essential Facts:

IV. Specific Major Problems:

V. Specific Sub-problems (if any):

VI. Proposed Solutions:

Immediate/Current

Long-Term

VII. Justification:

Case Scenario 19B

Rocky Valley University — Who's the Dr. Here?

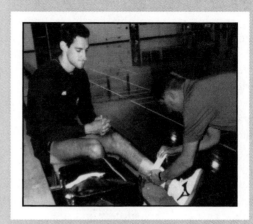

Ian Robertson's first year as Assistant Athletic Trainer at Rocky Valley University had been both rewarding and fulfilling, so he expected the upcoming year to be more of the same. Ian fondly recalls the day when he accepted the offer to join RVU's staff as Assistant Athletic Trainer and Clinical Instructor for the school's new CAAHEP (Commission on Accreditation of Allied Health Education Programs)-accredited undergraduate athletic training education program. Ian had been an NATA-BOC (National Athletic Trainers Association Board of Certification)-certified athletic trainer for 5 years and had been Head Athletic Trainer at a small community college before coming to Rocky Valley. Although he had enjoyed his former position, he would have the opportunity at Rocky Valley to teach students who aspired to become NATA-certified athletic trainers.

At RVU, Ian's clinical responsibilities included providing athletic training services for six intercollegiate athletic teams in addition to providing clinical supervision of the student athletic trainers assigned to work with those teams. He was required to be present at all scheduled practices and home competitions but was not required to travel to "away" competitions. Student athletic trainers traveled with their respective teams and provided athletic training services at "away" competition sites.

Ian's clinical skills were quickly recognized by his fellow athletic trainers, student athletic trainers, coaches, and student athletes. In addition, his professionalism, maturity, and teaching ability were noticed by all with whom he worked.

At the beginning of Ian's second year at Rocky Valley, Alex Sloan, the Head Athletic Trainer, redistributed the athletic team assignments for his staff. As a result of the new assignments, Ian found himself responsible for providing athletic training services for the women's varsity lacrosse team rather than the softball team, with whom he had enjoyed working the previous year. With the exception of this change, Ian's responsibilities remained basically the same. Upon being notified of the new assignment, Ian became anxious and concerned. He knew that Dr. Craig (PhD), the women's lacrosse coach, had a history of conflict with the athletic training staff. He had heard plenty of "horror stories" about Dr. Craig's confrontations with athletic trainers, his attempts to undermine the efforts of the athletic training staff, and his harsh treatment of injured athletes. Unfortunately, Dr. Craig was considered "an institution" at Rocky Valley, having led the women's lacrosse team to four national championships.

Dr. Craig had been brought to the university 8 years ago by Mr. Nicholson, RVU's Athletics Director, to revive a losing lacrosse program. Dr. Craig and Mr. Nicholson had played soccer together in college and had remained friends since their graduation. Therefore, Mr. Nicholson was familiar with Dr. Craig's past coaching success and did not hesitate to offer him the head coaching position at Rocky Valley immediately following the resignation of the former coach. Despite all he had heard about Dr. Craig, Ian was convinced that he could work successfully with the women's lacrosse team without conflict. Unfortunately, this was not to be so.

Throughout the lacrosse season Dr. Craig second-guessed Ian's decisions. He attempted to undermine Ian's (and the entire athletic staff's) credibility by openly criticizing, in front of his players, the athletic training staff and its work. Midway through the season, an incident occurred that resulted in Dr. Craig's refusing to even communicate with Ian for a week or more. During a game, one of the lacrosse players sustained a significant blow to the head. Ian's immediate evaluation following the injury revealed that the player had suffered a cerebral concussion and was not fit to return to participation. Dr. Craig argued vehemently for the player's return because she was the team's leading scorer and this was a critical conference game.

Dr. Craig was so intent on returning the player to the game that he threatened to use his influence at the college and in the community to have Ian fired if he refused to allow the player to return. Remaining calm, Ian ignored Dr. Craig's threat and explained his rationale for holding the player out of the game. The player did not return to play, and following the game, the university's team physician

confirmed Ian's evaluation and recommended 3 additional days of rest before returning to athletic participation.

The final lacrosse game of the season was an "away" game with traditional in-state rival, Sagewood College. As was customary, Ian called the certified athletic trainer at Sagewood and informed him that Annie, a student athletic trainer, would be accompanying the Rocky Valley team. He explained that Annie was not certified and had been instructed to ask for assistance if it was needed. Having made the necessary arrangements, he wished the team good luck as they loaded the bus for their trip.

As always, this year's Rocky Valley–Sagewood game was a close one, with the lead changing hands four times before halftime. The second half began with Rocky Valley down by two goals, but a quick score pulled them within one goal. As the celebrating players sprinted back toward midfield, everyone heard a chilling scream. One of Rocky Valley's players was on the ground holding her knee and screaming in pain. The officials quickly motioned to the Rocky Valley sideline for assistance, and both Annie and Dr. Craig sprinted toward the injured girl.

After calming the injured player, Annie was able to ascertain that she had planted her foot while running, and when she turned, she heard a "pop" and felt sharp pain in the knee. Just as Annie was about to examine the injured knee, Dr. Craig yelled, "Don't touch her! You're only a student. You don't know what you're doing." Startled by the outburst, Annie composed herself and confidently responded that she had gathered the necessary history and would like to continue her evaluation of the injury. Again Dr. Craig raised his voice: "Don't touch her. Just go back to the bench, and I'll take care of her." As Annie opened her mouth to respond, he loudly stated, "Look, I'm the doctor here, not you. I said I will take care of it."

Having observed the scene from her sideline, Sagewood's Head Athletic Trainer came onto the field, arriving on the scene just as

Annie was beginning to head back toward the bench. When the Sagewood trainer offered her assistance, Dr. Craig quickly and sternly told her to leave the player alone and "kindly return to the bench." Without examining the injured knee, Dr. Craig demanded that the injured player stand and get off the field. Obviously in a great deal of pain, the player limped, sobbing, to the bench. Annie applied an ice pack to the injury, but it did little to ease the pain.

Late that evening, Ian received a telephone call from the Sagewood trainer. She explained in great detail the events surrounding the injury to the Rocky Valley player. From information provided by Annie prior to the team's departure, she told Ian that she was quite certain the injury was serious and should be referred to an orthopedic specialist. Ian thanked her for her assistance and angrily hung up the phone.

Early the next morning, Ian contacted Annie, and they spoke at length about the incident. She told him everything, including how Dr. Craig had ordered her from the field and then "managed" the injury himself. Ian listened carefully and took written notes as she spoke. Not surprisingly, Annie's account of the events was practically identical to that provided by the Sagebrush athletic trainer the night before. Ian assured Annie that she had followed the proper protocol and told her that a situation like this would hopefully never happen again. That afternoon, Ian met with Alex Sloan and Rocky Valley's Athletics Director, Dr. Bolton.

Case Analysis Report Form
19B – Rocky Valley University — Who's the Dr. Here?

I. Brief Overview:

II. Principal Characters:

III. Essential Facts:

IV. Specific Major Problems:

V. Specific Sub-problems (if any):

VI. Proposed Solutions:

Immediate/Current

Long-Term

VII. Justification:

Case Scenario 19C

High Water High School — Caught Between a Rock and a Hard Place

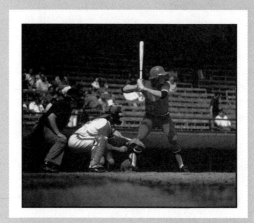

It is late spring at High Water High School. The weather is warm, the flowers are in bloom, and spring sports are nearing the end of their seasons. HWHS is a 4A school (2,500 students) with the luxury of having two certified athletic trainers. One of the athletic trainers, Bill Ball, is working today's home baseball game between High Water and conference rival Low Valley. Bill's major tasks are to monitor several players who will be playing with minor injuries, and to care for any injuries that might occur during the course of the game. A conference rule stipulates that Bill, as the host trainer, is also responsible for caring for injuries that players on the visiting team might sustain. Bill's responsibilities, however, do not include injury care for spectators and other non-athletes.

It's not that the Athletics Department does not recognize the possibility of spectator injuries. In fact, great care has been taken to design the playing facility in such a way as to protect spectators from injury. In addition to the 8-foot tall chainlink fence that completely surrounds the field, the only available spectator seating is directly behind home plate, extending about halfway down each baseline, and is protected by a 30-foot high wire-mesh backstop.

The weather at game time is hot and humid, and the competition is even hotter. The winner of this game will be the regular-season conference champion and will earn home-field advantage throughout the conference tournament. Going into the bottom of the ninth inning, HWHS is one run down. With the potential tying run on third base and one out, the batter hits a looping drive into short right field. The Low Valley right fielder charges the ball, dives, and makes a spectacular sliding catch. The third-base coach, assuming that the right fielder cannot regain his footing in time to make a good throw to the plate, sends the runner home. Surprisingly, the right fielder does a forward roll and comes up throwing. In a close play at the plate, the runner is called out. End of game.

The home fans are livid. Among them is the grandfather of the runner who was thrown out trying to score. He is obviously incensed. Screaming and yelling, his face is red with anger. Suddenly he becomes quiet and slumps back into his seat. People around him immediately begin yelling for help.

No medical personnel (doctor, EMS, etc.) are present, so Bill reacts instinctively. He tells the baseball coach to call 911. Bill is CPR-certified and had resuscitated a football player during a game this past season. By the time Bill reaches the stands, the man shows no signs of life. Bill checks for breathing — nothing. After giving two rescue breaths, he checks for a pulse — nothing. Without hesitation, Bill begins chest compressions. He asks bystanders if anyone is trained in CPR but gets no response. Without missing a beat, Bill continues his efforts — five compressions and one breath, five compressions and one breath.

The temperature seems to be getting hotter. "It must be at least 100 degrees," Bill thinks to himself. The welcome sound of a siren in the distance means that help is on the way. Shortly, the EMS crew takes over, frantically checking for a pulse. What had seemed like an eternity since the call to 911 was actually only 7 minutes.

As his grandfather was loaded into the ambulance, the young player thanked Bill for saving his life. As the ambulance pulled off, everyone was patting Bill on the back and congratulating him for another job well done. Bill was a hero — for a while. Unfortunately, the young player's grandfather was pronounced dead upon arrival at the local hospital. His brain had been deprived of oxygen for too long, and resuscitation attempts at the hospital were unsuccessful. Even though his compressions seemed to be sufficient to maintain blood flow, Bill's efforts apparently had been ineffective.

Two months after the incident, Bill received a certified letter. As he read it, he was devastated. He and the school were being sued by the deceased man's family for wrongful death resulting from negligence. As he tried to gather his thoughts, Bill wondered "What did I do? What didn't I do? What should I have done?"

Case Analysis Report Form
19C – High Water High School — Caught Between a Rock and a Hard Place

I. Brief Overview:

II. Principal Characters:

III. Essential Facts:

IV. Specific Major Problems:

V. Specific Sub-problems (if any):

VI. Proposed Solutions:

Immediate/Current

Long-Term

VII. Justification:

Case Scenario 19D

Slippery Slope University — Hey, Who Needs Another Policy?

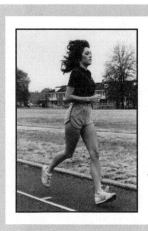

Jason Long has been an athletic trainer for 5 years at Slippery Slope University (SSU). During that time, one of Jason's primary assignments has been working with the men's and women's cross-country teams. The teams train year-round with their primary competition in the fall and some minor competition scheduled in the spring. Because the athletes are busy year-round, Jason is busy year-round. He works with the athletes on their workout schedules, both running and weight training, and advises them on their diet for training and competition. He is particularly conscious of overuse injuries and does not hesitate to inform the cross-country coach, Mike Thomas, when he thinks the athletes are at their limit.

Like most athletic trainers, Jason has developed a close working relationship with his athletes. He knows their habits, and he knows when they are up and when they are down. Recently Jason has become concerned about several of the female runners and the amount of weight they have been losing. He is particularly concerned about Stephanie Lee, a junior runner who is 5' 7" and weighs barely 100 pounds. It is August, and the competitive season will be starting in about a month. When the spring

term ended in May, Stephanie weighed 125 pounds. Jason does not consider himself an expert on anorexia nervosa, but he has been doing quite a bit of reading lately on the anorexic female athlete triad: disordered eating, amenorrhea, and osteoporosis.

Jason has heard Stephanie talking about her weight on many occasions, in which she has indicated that if she did not weigh so much, she probably could do better in the upcoming competitions. Jason also has noticed that Stephanie's maximum weight lifted this fall was noticeably lower than what she had been lifting the previous fall. Jason had asked Stephanie about this on several occasions, and she had told him she was just fighting off a bug.

When he talks to her about her weight, she says there is no problem. When he finally decides to ask her whether she is having her periods, she tells him, "Not that it's any of your business, but I haven't had a regular period since I began running seriously in the eleventh grade."

Jason is really concerned now. He believes that if he does not do something, Stephanie's condition will only get worse, and when competition begins, she is likely to experience stress fractures or worse. He contacts Coach James about taking Stephanie off the team temporarily and getting her to see a physician about her possible eating disorder. Coach James says he sees no problem. Stephanie's times have been just fine in practice. Besides, he thinks that if Stephanie is having any problem, she will see a doctor on her own.

Knowing that this is not likely to happen, Jason seeks advice from the head trainer, Miles Kelly. Miles informs Jason that the athletic department has no policy regarding athletes and anorexia and he sees no way to take Stephanie off the team. Jason says there should be a policy. This should be considered no different from any other injury that would preclude an athlete's participation in an event. Miles agrees and sets up an appointment with the athletic director, George Goble.

When Jason and Miles arrive for the meeting, the first thing George says is, "Bring me up to speed on anorexia. I'm not sure I know everything I need to know. And tell me why you think this young woman has anorexia."

Jason gives George the limited information he has on anorexia and tells him what he has observed in Stephanie. He also tells George what he thinks the outcome might be if no one intervenes.

When he is finished, George replies, "What you're telling me is that you suspect this young woman is exercising herself into a state of anorexia — and probably not eating like she should either. And if she continues this, she might have stress fractures or more serious health problems."

Jason answers in the affirmative and George continues, "And what you think we should do is come up with some policy that will allow you to recommend she be taken off the team until she is examined by a physician who has some expertise in eating disorders.

And the physician will either clear her to return to the team or recommend some kind of intervention?"

Again Jason replies in the affirmative and adds that he believes there certainly will be a liability situation if anything should happen to Stephanie, especially because the athletic department, through its trainers, have done nothing to prevent it.

George then says, "This liability thing is just what I've been thinking about. What if we take Stephanie off the team and she chooses not to see a physician? We can't make her see a doctor. What if she leaves the team and continues to exercise and ends up having all these problems anyway? What if she is out running by herself and collapses? Couldn't we be liable for that? After all, we ran her off the team. Wouldn't she be better off on the team if something like that happens? There would be someone there to get her assistance, and she would be more likely to recover.

"If we have a policy on anorexia, we'll be setting ourselves up for problems. We'll have female athletes making claims against us for harassment and discrimination. It will be better for us not to have a policy and let this be something for the athlete and her family to work through. No. We will not have a policy on anorexia."

Jason and Miles leave George's office and return to the training room. As they talk about the situation, they cannot decide what to do next. Should they talk to the team physician? Should they set up an appointment with a counselor at the wellness center? Should they contact Stephanie's parents? Should they go over George's head and talk to someone in administration — maybe the Dean of Students or even the President? They feel strongly that something should be done, but they are not certain what the next step should be.

Case Analysis Report Form
19D – Slippery Slope University — Hey, Who Needs Another Policy?

I. Brief Overview:

II. Principal Characters:

III. Essential Facts:

IV. Specific Major Problems:

V. Specific Sub-problems (if any):

VI. Proposed Solutions:

   Immediate/Current

   Long-Term

VII. Justification:

Case Analysis Activities: Health Promotion and Adult Fitness

20

Case Scenario 20A

Fancy Fred's Fri-Daddy, Inc. — Well, It Was a Good Idea!

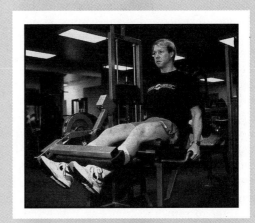

Fancy Fred's Fri-Daddy, Inc. is one of the region's largest and most successful fast-food franchise corporations, and home of the world famous "Fancy Fred's Fri-Daddy Deluxe Burger Basket." Like all other companies, Fancy Fred's is interested in ways to cut costs and increase profit. So, when the company's group medical insurance representative said the company could save money by establishing an employee wellness program, Fred Ford, company CEO, was anxious to give it a try.

John Pitts, a recent graduate of nearby Blakedale State University, was selected to head up the new employee wellness program. John had a degree in exercise science

and was an honor graduate. In addition to his academic credentials, he was popular among his fellow students and professors and eager to begin his new job at Fancy Fred's corporate headquarters.

John discovered that company had three vice presidents who reported directly to Mr. Ford. The vice president in charge of the wellness program was Mr. Treblehorn, Vice President for Personnel Services. This was the logical arrangement, as the wellness program was viewed as an employee benefit. John enjoyed working under Mr. Treblehorn because he was given free rein to run the program as he thought best. The only constraint was a rather meager budget. Mr.

Treblehorn, however, explained to John that the wellness program was a bit of an experimental program. If it proved to be cost-effective, he could expect a significant increase in his operating budget.

John's first task was to determine the type of organizational plan that would be best for the program. His first weeks on the job were spent surveying employees to determine what types of activities they wanted, scheduling and teaching classes — doing everything that had to be done to make the program successful. He soon decided that he needed an assistant, someone who could help with administrative duties and teach many of the classes. After reviewing his budget, John discovered that he could afford to hire only a part-time assistant.

As he was exploring the possibility of hiring a part-time assistant, John received a disturbing memo from Mr. Treblehorn. According to the memo, the group medical insurance carrier had determined that Fancy Fred's wellness program would have to increase employee participation by at least 30% to qualify for the lower premium rates the company had promised. John realized that, even with a part-time assistant, increasing participation by 30% would be virtually impossible.

If he could just find a way to hire a full-time assistant, maybe, just maybe, he could meet the insurance company's expectations. He considered the possibility of shifting money from other budget areas so he could hire a full-time assistant. After all, he had a little extra money in the budget that he had been saving for a small publicity campaign and a piece or

two of badly needed equipment. He decided to schedule a meeting with Mr. Treblehorn to discuss the dilemma and possibly request additional money.

During their meeting, Mr. Treblehorn approved John's proposal to shift funds from other budget areas for the purpose of hiring a full-time assistant. He advised John, however, that additional budgetary funding could not be made available, as the original point of starting the wellness program was to lower company expenditures, not increase them. He stated that increasing the wellness program budget at this time simply would not be cost-effective.

John acknowledged his understanding of the company's position and said he would explore other ways to solve the problem. The meeting concluded with a request from Mr. Treblehorn that John report back to him in 2 weeks concerning his progress on the matter.

Although John found Mr. Treblehorn easy to talk to, he had provided little help in resolving the budgetary dilemma. To make matters worse, the day after his meeting with Mr. Treblehorn, John received a memo from Mr. Ford stating that the company's group medical insurance company had announced an increase in the minimum number of wellness program participants necessary to continue receiving lower premium rates. Now John was faced with the decision of how to use what funds he did have. Should he proceed with hiring an assistant so more activities could be offered? Should he launch a publicity effort to attract more employees to participate in the program? Or, should he — ?

Case Analysis Report Form
20A – Fancy Fred's Fri-Daddy, Inc. — Well, It Was a Good Idea!

   I. Brief Overview:

  II. Principal Characters:

 III. Essential Facts:

IV. Specific Major Problems:

V. Specific Sub-problems (if any):

VI. Proposed Solutions:

Immediate/Current

Long-Term

VII. Justification:

Case Scenario 20B

Wellness World — New Kid in Town

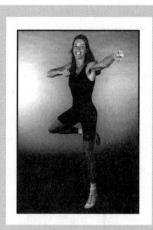

Wellness World was one of many fitness clubs in Metro City, a city of 250,000. Although busy from opening until closing (7 a.m. to 10 p.m., Monday through Saturday), the facility was significantly understaffed. Dick, the manager, and Susan, the assistant manager, were the only full-time employees, and most of the teaching was done by six part-time fitness instructors. Therefore, when Jane walked through the door looking for a job, she seemed almost too good to be true.

Jane was new to Metro City. A beautiful blonde with a master's degree in physical education, she was a single mother of a 6-year old son. Her resume indicated that she had 5 years' experience as a fitness instructor in another state. Everything about Jane was just perfect — almost. During her interview, Jane told Dick that she could work only from 9 a.m. to 5 p.m., and no weekends. Dick was so impressed by Jane's experience and appearance that he saw little need to contact her references, and offered her the position on the spot. She happily accepted and became Wellness World's first full-time instructor.

Less than a month after Jane started work, her young son got sick at school. When his teacher called Jane at work, she immediately clocked out and went home early. Susan, the assistant manager, immediately called Bart, one of the part-time instructors, to come in early. Bart was happy to get in a few extra hours.

Everything was working out fine until Jane began to miss work often. Each time she failed to show up or had to leave early, Bart was called in to take her place. At first he enjoyed the opportunities to make a little extra money. As time went by, though, he became more than just a little aggravated at being interrupted during his days off.

One day Jane approached Dick and asked for a raise. After all, she reasoned, her graduate degree and previous experience certainly justified a better salary than she was making. Also, with a young child to care for, she needed to make more money.

Dick mentioned Jane's request to Susan and asked her opinion. Susan was somewhat perplexed. On one hand, she had noticed on several occasions that Jane did not seem to have much knowledge about the fitness business. On the other hand, since Dick had surely checked her references, Jane knew he would have never hired Jane if she was not well qualified. Susan told Dick she wasn't sure that a raise was a good idea but, as manager, he should make the decision.

Dick decided to give Jane a substantial raise, fearing that otherwise she might quit and move to another club. When the part-time instructors learned of Jane's raise, they were furious. Bart mentioned their feelings to Dick and was told that Jane deserved a raise. Furthermore, if any of the part-time instructors had a problem with it, they were welcome to find somewhere else to work.

After receiving her raise, Jane's absences became even more frequent. As usual, Susan relied on Bart to "take up the slack," even though his hourly salary was barely that of Jane's. One day Bart and Jane were working at the same time, and he decided to confront her about her frequent absences.

"I thought you would be thankful for the extra work," Jane angrily replied.

Bart exploded, "@#&%&% ^$*&#@% !!!" At that moment, Dick came into the room, just in time to hear Bart's outburst. He told the two that, though he was unaware that there had been a problem, he tended to agree with Jane. Still angry, Bart clocked out and left for the evening.

The next morning when Bart reported for work, Dick called him into his office to discuss what had happened the day before. Bart told his side of the story. Dick shook his head and said, "I understand how you must feel, but I'm not sure what I should do."

Case Analysis Report Form
20B – Wellness World — New Kid in Town

I. Brief Overview:

II. Principal Characters:

III. Essential Facts:

IV. Specific Major Problems:

V. Specific Sub-problems (if any):

VI. Proposed Solutions:

Immediate/Current

Long-Term

VII. Justification:

Case Scenario 20C

Seagull Performance Systems, Inc. — Will Someone Please Tell Me What To Do?

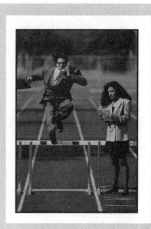

Alex Arlington is the Director of Wellness at Seagull Performance Systems, Inc. When Alex accepted the position 10 years ago, the wellness program was little more than a small room with one treadmill, one stationary bicycle, and one employee — Alex.

Alex's first administrative decision was to hire Shirley Pawlsen as his secretary. Shirley was a bright young lady with exceptional clerical and organizational skills. In her first 2 weeks on the job, Shirley set up an efficient filing system, designed a master schedule for all of Alex's appointments, and greeted Alex each morning with a cup of coffee in one hand and important messages (in priority order) and the day's calendar in the other. Not long thereafter, colleagues began to good-naturedly refer to Shirley as the "Executive Director" of the program, to which Alex always replied, "You're just jealous."

Over the past 10 years, the wellness program experienced tremendous popularity, success, and growth. The program now is located in a newly completed 30,000-square-foot facility complete with aerobics room, weight room, three racquetball courts, indoor pool, walk-jog track, and showering/dressing facilities. In addition to Alex and Shirley, there are four full-time employees: Pam, the wellness educator; Stan, the exercise physiologist; Karen, the fitness coordinator; and Rod, the aquatics coordinator. Alex could not be happier.

Alex's contract allows him 4 weeks of vacation, which he usually takes a few days at a time throughout the year. This year, however, Alex and his wife took the vacation they had always dreamed of — a 3-week trip to Europe. What a wonderful vacation it was. Alex was able to put work completely out of his mind, although he frequently remarked, "We could never have done this if Shirley wasn't 'minding the store.'"

When Alex reported for work the first morning after returning from vacation, he was shocked — to put it mildly. When he reached the wellness facility, there was no cup of coffee, no daily calendar, and, worst of all, no Shirley! The day after Alex and his wife left for Europe, Shirley suffered a stroke. She was rushed to the local hospital, where her condition worsened. The decision was made to transfer her to a major medical center several hundreds of miles away. The good news was that Shirley's prognosis was positive. The bad news was that she would never be able to return to work. The stroke had damaged her memory and left her (temporarily, it was hoped) unable to communicate. Needless to say, Alex was devastated.

When Alex opened the door to his office, he experienced his second shock. His desk was piled with messages, memos, and mail, the message light on his telephone was blinking, and, upon checking his computer, he found numerous e-mail messages. After discarding all the junk mail and insignificant messages, Alex still had many communications that would require his attention. The problem was, what should he do first? Second? Third? And so on. "Oh, Shirley," he muttered, "I never realized how much I depended on you. Where do I even begin?"

The following are some of the communications requiring Alex's action. How should he prioritize them? What about other issues?

Voice-Mail Message

Mon., 6/19/98, 11:20 am

Alex,

Call me ASAP concerning your request for funds to modify the swimming pool in your facility. I'm afraid a big mistake has been made. When you were notified in May that the money was available, the request had not received Davidson's signature of approval. Now, I am embarrassed to say, your request has been denied by the "people at the top." Good news though . . . I will see that money for the pool upgrade is set aside in next year's budget. Hope this doesn't cause a problem.

Emily Conyers, ext. 258
Accounting Department

Telephone Message

TO _Alex_   DATE _6/28/98_   TIME _3:30 pm_

While you were out _Susan Hardy of Dynakleen_ called.

She's really upset! Says they submitted the low bid for reconditioning the upholstery on the weight machines, but NuSeats got the contract. Wants to know what's going on. Says if she doesn't hear from you within 48 hrs, she's going to talk to their lawyers about a lawsuit.

Inter-Office Memo

TO: Alex Arlington
FROM: Sonya Jackson
RE: Lack of Minority Personnel
DATE: June 16, 1998

The Employee Welfare Committee is concerned about the diminishing numbers of minority employees in many departments. It has been brought to our attention that, as the result of the transfer of Eugene Porter to Human Resources, the Wellness Program currently has no minority staff members.

Since nearly 40% of our total company workforce is made up of minority employees, and many of these participate in the Wellness Program, we believe that the ethnic composition of your staff should be representative of those the program is designed to serve.

Please get tin touch with me immediately so we can discuss this issue prior to our July 15 meeting.

    cc: C. Withers, Vice President
         Human Resources

E-Mail Message

TO: arlingab@spsinc.com
FROM: ulmberg@spsinc.com
TOPIC: Annual Combined-Charities Fund Drive
DATE: June 21, 1998

Hey Alex,

Don't forget we have a luncheon meeting on Tuesday, July 3, to report on your department's role in this year's campaign. As per our June 10 conversation, you and your staff will be in charge of this year's kick-off event to be held September 4. Please bring a list of tentative activities.

Thanks,
Karl

County Department of Public Health

June 12, 1998

Mr. Alex Arlington
Wellness Director
Seagull Performance Systems
Your City, USA

Dear Mr. Arlington:

Our office has been informed that an inspector from the State Department of Occupational Safety and Health will be visiting your facility on Thursday, July 5, to inspect your swimming pool and shower and bathroom facilities for compliance with the revised regulations on water safety standards in a public facility.

You should note that, although your facility passed its initial inspection just prior to its official opening, the filtration system in place at the time is no longer acceptable according to the new standards. In the event that you have not replaced the original system, you must contact the SDOSH office no later than June 28 to request a delay in the scheduled inspection visit. You may wish to do this anyway, since failure to meet any of the new standards could result in your facility being closed down until necessary changes can be made.

I will be leaving on vacation on July 1. However, if you have any questions prior to that time, please feel free to call on me.

Have a nice day!

Sincerely,

Raymond P. Fawcett
County Health Commissioner

Note: This scenario was adapted from "The Administrative In-Basket: A Simulated Exercise" in *Creative Administration in Physical Education and Athletics*, by R. A. Pestolesi and W. A. Sinclair (Englewood Cliffs, NJ: Prentice-Hall, 1978).

Case Analysis Report Form
20C – Seagull Performance Systems, Inc. — Will Someone Please Tell Me What To Do?

I. Brief Overview:

II. Principal Characters:

III. Essential Facts:

IV. Specific Major Problems:

V. Specific Sub-problems (if any):

VI. Proposed Solutions:

    Immediate/Current

    Long-Term

VII. Justification:

Case Scenario 20D

Live Better By Sweating Fitness Center — A Testy Dilemma

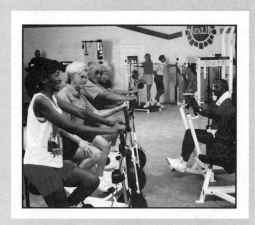

George Alexander is a fitness expert at Live Better By Sweating Fitness Center (LBBS), affectionately known as the Sweat Box. George has been working at the Sweat Box for 5¹/₂ years. Like all other full-time employees at LBBS, George is on an annual contract. His major responsibilities are the development and supervision of fitness programs for clients who come to the Sweat Box to improve their fitness levels and lose weight. George works primarily with male clients between the ages of 50 and 60 years. His clients view George as somewhat of a specialist in the area of heart-attack prevention, as he has not lost a client at the Sweat Box. This is an especially good record because George tends to get highly unfit clients.

While George was in his undergraduate program at Old South University, he completed a semester-long internship in the cardiac rehabilitation unit at Major Medical Hospital (MMH), a state-supported teaching hospital. He has maintained a close relationship with some of the cardiac specialists at the hospital. Because of this relationship, the cardiac specialists refer a number of their clients to George at LBBS. Because LBBS is not a cardiac rehabilitation center,

the referrals are only people who have complained of chest pains, undergone a stress test and angiogram, and been classified as having low to medium risk for heart attack. These patients have some minor cardiac arterial blockage, but the physicians believe the best way to deal with these patients is through diet and exercise.

George's record is about to change. A new client has just joined the Sweat Box. He is 55-year old Jamie Smits. Jamie is 50 pounds overweight, smokes 1¹/₂ packs of cigarettes per day, and the only exercise he gets is working to keep his son off his back about not exercising. Jamie eats lunch every day at the Old Town Restaurant, where he typically orders the fat burger special with french fries and washes it all down with a couple of beers.

When Jamie joined LBBS, he told the club health education specialist, Megan Troy, that he was joining LBBS specifically to work with George. (Jamie's son had known George in college and had told his dad that "He da man!") Jamie was apparently aware of George's relationship with the cardiac specialists at MMH and talked about them extensively as Megan took his medical history and had him complete several questionnaires concerning his diet and exercise habits.

Part of the health interview by Megan, who is finishing her third year as a full-time employee at LBBS, included a clearance for exercise form that Megan was authorized to complete for clients under age 35 with no history of cardiac abnormalities. But the form had to be completed by the client's physician if the client was older than 35 or had some history of cardiac difficulty. Jamie had informed Megan that he had no history of cardiac difficulty yet. Megan inadvertently checked the clearance box and signed the form. Jamie also signed a participation agreement indicating that he was aware of the nature of the program and that his state of health would cause no problems in participation.

Megan then sent Jamie to see Liz Rubble, a registered nurse, who moonlights part-time at the Sweat Box when she is not working full-time at MMH. Liz's job was to draw blood and send it off to be analyzed for cholesterol levels. Liz informed Jamie of the procedure, gave him a form explaining how the blood was to be drawn, where it would be sent for analysis (to MMH), what it would be analyzed for, and how the results were to be used. After several questions to ensure that the blood would be analyzed for cholesterol only, Jamie signed the forms. Liz informed Jamie that for the test to be valid, it could be taken only after a 12-hour fasting period. Jamie said he understood, and a time was scheduled the next evening for the blood test.

Jamie came in the next evening, saw Liz for the blood draw, and was sent back to Megan. Megan reviewed some of the information collected from the previous day. She told Jamie that his health profile indicated that he was a good match for the program. She explained the locus of control scale he had completed and told him that he was externally controlled. She told him that George had his best results working with externals because they were more willing to follow instructions and were more faithful in their attendance.

Jamie was pumped. Finally someone was saying something positive about who he was and predicting some success for him. But he would have to wait a while because George's next class of newcomers would not get started for 2 more weeks.

Megan gave Jamie a diet guide and told him that while George was handling the exercise, she would be conducting nutrition education classes covering the material in the guide. She also informed Jamie that his blood analysis would be back and that the significance of the readings would be covered in the class. She let him know that the cholesterol readings were confidential and no one's cholesterol levels would be disclosed in class unless individual clients would choose to do that on their own. Megan set his appointment for George's class in 2 weeks and told Jamie that he should read the diet guide before then. Megan told Jamie that George's first class would be a "get to know you" session in which he would tell the clients what the class involves and the type of clothing and shoes they would need.

A week later George is going over Jamie's history, taken by Megan, to familiarize himself with who will be coming in. As he reads Jamie's records, he notes that even though Jamie is 55, Megan had signed his clearance form. Megan is off the day George is reading Jamie's records, so he makes a note to ask her about the discrepancy and paper-clips it to Jamie's folder.

That same day, Jamie's blood results arrive at LBBS. When Liz comes in that evening, she collects the blood analysis reports and prepares to place them in the individual client's folder. Liz follows a procedure established by the owner of the Sweat Box. She examines the report and makes notes on any readings that might indicate a serious problem, such as extremely high LDL readings or extremely low HDL readings. She shares this information with Megan and George, and they devise a strategy for dealing with each client. A copy of the strategy is placed in the client's folder.

When Liz opens Jamie's report, she is surprised to find two forms instead of the usual one. Jamie's blood seems to have been analyzed for something more than cholesterol. MMH requires all of its employees to take an initial drug test when they are hired and then to take an annual test thereafter. Someone inadvertently had run the MMH employee drug test on Jamie's blood. The test showed positive for cocaine.

Being a nurse, Liz is familiar with the relationship between cocaine and cardiac arrhythmias. She believes this poses a risk for Jamie as he enters an exercise program, especially since he is a 55-year-old, overweight smoker. She thinks she must tell George but then remembers that there was no permission to perform a drug test on Jamie's blood. If they tell Jamie he cannot be in the exercise program, he will want to know why. They will either have to disclose the mistake or manufacture a reason. Liz decides she has to tell George.

When George gets the news, he says, "I'm not surprised. I knew his son in college. He was always whacked out on something. It apparently runs in the family." Liz thinks this is a little extreme but does not say anything. She just wants to know what George is going to do with the information. George says that there is really no reason to let anyone know anything. He thinks the initial phase of the program is low enough not to cause Jamie any problem and he (George) will monitor Jamie closely to make sure he is okay. There is no need to get the guys at the blood lab at MMH into trouble. George apparently has forgotten the note he had put on Jamie's file.

A week goes by, and Jamie shows up for the first class. Everything goes fine and plans are made for the group (which has six new clients) to report back the next evening for their first exercise session. As luck would have it, the next day on the way to the Sweat Box, Jamie notices a slight tightness in his chest. When he gets to the exercise room, he informs George. George takes Jamie's pulse and finds it beating faster than he would expect, even for someone in Jamie's condition. He decides to take Jamie's blood pressure and finds that it is only slightly elevated. George decides that Jamie is just a little uptight about beginning the program and tells him to join the other clients.

George has his clients walk on the treadmill for a few minutes at a pace slightly faster than a normal walk to warm up a little before he puts them through a stretching routine. He explains this to the clients and starts each one separately to ensure that they are walking with no problems. Jamie happens to be the first up. George gets him started and moves to the next client. As George is getting to the last client, he hears a groan and a thud. When he looks around, Jamie is face down on the treadmill. Luckily, the safety clip has stopped the treadmill.

George rushes to Jamie, turns him over, and checks for a pulse. Finding none, he immediately starts CPR and calls for Liz. As she appears, he tells her to call 911. She does and then returns to assist George. She can feel a pulse as George makes the compressions, but when he stops, there is nothing. George continues CPR, assisted by Liz.

EMS arrives in a short time and manages to establish a baseline heart rate. As they are getting Jamie ready for transport, George tells the EMT to be sure to have Jamie's blood tested when they get him to the emergency room because there is a good chance he is on cocaine.

It is 2 weeks later, and Jamie has survived a heart attack caused by a 95% blockage in a lower branch of his right anterior artery that apparently was closed by a small thrombosis. Quick action in the emergency room had prevented the need for open-heart surgery. Medication administered there had dissolved the clot. Jamie has undergone angioplasty and had a stint placed in his right anterior artery to keep it open. He will be under close observation by the cardiac specialists at MMH for the next 6 months. If he makes it through that period, his prognosis is good — provided he loses weight, stops smoking, gets his cholesterol down, and starts to exercise moderately.

The primary problem Jamie has now is that his insurance company will not pay his hospital bills. The health insurance policy has a drug clause stipulating that no payment will be made for any health problem brought about as a result of addiction to drugs. It should be pointed out that no drug test was ever taken in the emergency room the night Jamie had his heart attack.

And what's going on at LBBS? Bubba Sweat, the owner/operator, has fired George and Megan, claiming that their actions, and their actions alone, were responsible for the incident that nearly cost Jamie his life. Liz still has her part-time job.

Case Analysis Report Form
20D – Live Better By Sweating Fitness Center — A Testy Dilemma

I. Brief Overview:

II. Principal Characters:

III. Essential Facts:

IV. Specific Major Problems:

V. Specific Sub-problems (if any):

VI. Proposed Solutions:

Immediate/Current

Long-Term

VII. Justification:

Case Analysis Activities: Recreation and Intramural Activities

Case Scenario 21A

Brockington College — You Try to be a Nice Guy . . .

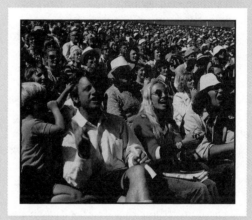

About 4 months before completing the coursework for his master's degree in recreation, Rex Cars applied for the position of Director of Intramurals at nearby Brockington College. Upon interviewing for the position, Rex found out that the school has just built four high-rise dormitories. This was a significant event, as Brockington had never before had on-campus housing for students. Located in a major urban area, most of the college's students would continue to be commuters.

Although he had no experience as an intramural director, Rex had been actively involved in intramural sports in college, and also had played on recreation teams while he was in the Air Force. Despite his lack of administrative experience, the college was eager to hire him and even offered to allow him to complete his master's thesis while working at the college. Rex was excited about the opportunity and accepted the position.

Rex's excitement was tempered by his lack of knowledge about intramural administration. While in graduate school, however, he had worked as an assistant in the County Recreation Department, so he did have some administrative experience. His duties had included responsibility for several youth sports leagues, such as team assignments, coaching appointments, equipment management, scheduling, and record-keeping.

Upon arrival at Brockington, Rex and his wife moved into a new apartment, which the college provided as part of his contract. He soon discovered that the "intramural program" that preceded his arrival was actually a loosely organized fraternity program of Greek Athletics. The Greek Athletics program had been under the direction of the college's Athletics Department, and under the supervision of the Director of Athletics, Marilyn Rozarro. Five fraternities competed in flag football and basketball, with championship points awarded according to each fraternity's standing in each sport.

Rex had no idea how serious the fraternities were about the Greek Athletics program, but he was about to find out. Dr. Rozarro suggested that Rex create a Greek division in the new intramural program, and that the schedule be designed so the perennial powers from the Greek division would meet in the final regular season game. Rex thought this sounded like a great idea.

Rex encountered his first problem when he scheduled a team captains' meeting, at which time he planned to introduce the new intramural program format. The Greeks were not the least bit enthusiastic about playing in the new intramural program, especially when the flag football schedule was to start the same weekend as the traditional Greek Alumni Games. They also complained that Rex's idea of limiting rosters to 16 players (8 players on the field at one time) discriminated against the fraternities, which typically had 35 to 40 players on their rosters. Because this was his first year on the job, Rex agreed to delay the start of the schedule and allow unlimited roster size so he could win the cooperation of the fraternities.

The flag football program began the week after the Greek Alumni Games — which, incidentally, drew more spectators than the school's varsity football team. The intramural league was made up of the five Greek teams

and five independent teams. It soon became obvious that the Greek teams were much stronger than the independent teams.

As the season progressed, Rex's greatest challenge was finding officials for the games. In previous years the fraternities had provided their own officials. But without the fraternity officials, Rex was often forced to officiate many of the games himself. This made supervision difficult, as two games were played simultaneously on separate fields. Rex did arrange to have an athletic trainer at each game.

During the third week of the season, the undefeated independent team was scheduled to play one of the stronger Greek teams. On the other field, the independent team did not have enough players, so the game was declared a forfeit. Therefore, Rex assigned all the officials to work the remaining game. As Rex was putting away the equipment from the forfeit game, he was approached by the Greek members winning by forfeit, wanting to play a practice game because they had not had the opportunity to play. Rex stated that it was fine with him, but they asked him to officiate. He reluctantly agreed, and the practice game proceeded.

The game seemed to go off without a hitch until Rex was walking off the field afterward. The captain of the fraternity team came to him and told him that Jack (one of his players) had been taken to a hospital. Surprised, Rex asked what had happened. He was told that the player was kicked in the groin early in the second half. Rex could not recall seeing any unusual collision but did remember that Jack did not play most of the second half.

Rex contacted the athletic trainer who had worked the day's games and was told that she had evaluated Jack immediately following the injury. She reported that he had complained of abdominal pain, so she took him to the training room. On the way in, Jack had collapsed but quickly regained consciousness. The athletic trainer summoned campus police, who took Jack to hospital. She assured Rex that she felt certain the injury was not particularly serious.

Assuming that everything that could be done had been done, Rex and his wife left for a weekend visit at the home of his parents.

As he walked to his office Monday morning, Rex was met by the captain of the fraternity team. When Rex asked him what was wrong, the student swallowed hard and said, "They gave Jack his last rites last night." Apparently the kick had ruptured Jack's colon, resulting in a massive abdominal infection. Later in the week, Rex was sitting in his apartment, when there was knock on the door. Rex opened the door to face the college's Dean of Students. He knew what had happened. Jack had died.

Almost 1 year to the day after the accident, Rex received notice that he and the school were being sued for negligence.

Case Analysis Report Form
21A – Brockington College — You Try to be a Nice Guy —

I. Brief Overview:

II. Principal Characters:

III. Essential Facts:

IV. Specific Major Problems:

V. Specific Sub-problems (if any):

VI. Proposed Solutions:

Immediate/Current

Long-Term

VII. Justification:

Case Scenario 21B

Walston State University — Who Said Anything About Being Fair?

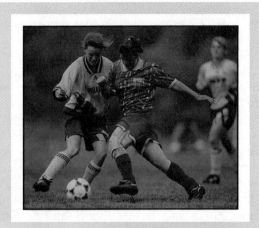

They simply did not think it was fair — not fair at all! "They" were the members of the Walston State University women's soccer team. The spring semester had just begun, and the soccer team was getting dressed for practice when Kellie Reynolds, the team captain, announced that the women's lacrosse team had been invited to compete in the National Championship Tournament in March. When asked, Kellie said she had gotten the news from a sign posted outside the Recreational Sports office, announcing a "reorganization meeting for the women's lacrosse team." Having played on the lacrosse team along with her soccer teammates during the fall semester, Kellie was surprised to learn of the post-season invitation — and even more surprised that a new team would be formed to represent the university in the tournament.

"That's just not fair," said Tammy Roper. "We made that team what it was, and now we don't get to play for the championship."

"You're right," added Kellie. "Without us the team wouldn't have won the conference championship. And without that, there would be no championship tournament invitation. And no, because it's soccer season, we can't

play in the tournament. I know — why don't we ask coach? Maybe she'll agree."

"Yeah, right," said Tammy, dejected.

In the fall semester, Walston State decided to add women's lacrosse to its intercollegiate athletics program. It was decided, however, that the first year the sport would be introduced as a club sport with no affiliation with NCAA. After all, the school had not even hired a coach, much less begun to recruit players. So members of the women's soccer team had thought that playing lacrosse would be both fun and a good way to get in shape for the soccer season. As Coach York, the soccer coach, was not familiar with the physical nature of lacrosse, she endorsed the idea of her players' participation.

Unfortunately, two of the soccer players were injured playing lacrosse, and both required surgery. Although Coach York was not happy about the prospect of additional injuries, she allowed her players to complete the lacrosse season with one stipulation: After the initial season, soccer players would not be allowed to play lacrosse in the future. After all, the soccer players were receiving grant-in-aid money for playing soccer, not lacrosse.

Unexpectedly, the first-year lacrosse team not only breezed through its conference schedule with an undefeated record, but it easily won the conference championship. Many of the soccer players actually enjoyed playing lacrosse more than playing soccer. Kellie and some of the other players approached Mr. Marvel, the Director of Athletics, with a proposal: "If we each agree to sign a release form stating that if we are injured playing lacrosse, we will forfeit our soccer grant-in-aid money, could we then continue to play both lacrosse and soccer?"

Coach Marvel did not even need to think about it. His answer was a quick and definite "No!"

Without the soccer players, Mr. Gordon, the Director of Intramural and Recreational Sports, was stuck. The National Championship Tournament was out of the question. Officials from the National Lacrosse Organization (NLO), however, noted that Walston State had signed a contract agreeing to field a team in return for the NLO's financial and developmental instruction support. So where was he going to find players? NLO officials suggested a team reorganization meeting.

Several girls showed up for the meeting — many of whom were known to be good athletes. Many were also good friends of the soccer players who had played on the lacrosse team in the fall. This posed a problem. After attending the reorganization meeting and stating their interest in playing, none of them showed up for the first two practice sessions. When Mr. Gordon contacted the soccer players to ask them for their lacrosse uniforms, he was met with three angry words: "It's not fair!" Now he knew why his "new" players had not followed through with their intentions to play.

What now?

Case Analysis Report Form
21B – "Walston State University — Who Said Anything About Being Fair?"

I. Brief Overview:

II. Principal Characters:

III. Essential Facts:

IV. Specific Major Problems:

V. Specific Sub-problems (if any):

VI. Proposed Solutions:

Immediate/Current

Long-Term

VII. Justification:

Case Analysis Report Form
21C – Clifton Community College — When It Rains, It Pours

I. Brief Overview:

II. Principal Characters:

III. Essential Facts:

IV. Specific Major Problems:

V. Specific Sub-problems (if any):

VI. Proposed Solutions:

Immediate/Current

Long-Term

VII. Justification:

Case Scenario 21D

North Star Technical College — Anyone For a Little Game of Basketball?

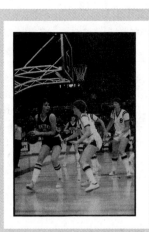

North Star Technical College has one of the finest intramural sports programs anywhere — thanks, in large part, to the hard work of Intramural Director Sandi James. Sandi has developed a well-organized program, with competition in more than 20 different sports and activities. More North Star Tech students participated in intramurals than in the school's intercollegiate sports program.

One of the main rules of the college's intramural program is that any student who has played a sport on a college varsity team is ineligible to participate in that same sport in the intramural program. The former athlete, however, may participate in any of the other intramural activities. This rule applies to all former players, regardless of how little or how much they had played or the level (NAIA, NCAA-III, NCAA-II, or NCAA-I) at which they had played.

Just before intramural basketball season, a student, Judy Byers, approached Ms. James, seeking assistance in joining a team. Because Sandi was unfamiliar with the young lady, she assumed her to be a first-year (freshman or transfer) student on campus and agreed to help her find a team whose roster was not full.

At the end of the first evening of basketball competition, Sandi was walking out of the gym when she was confronted by three girls. Their team had lost its opening game earlier in the evening, and they were upset about their opponents having used an ineligible player. They went on to explain that the player in question was ineligible because she had played on the school's varsity basketball team. When they identified the ineligible player as Judy Byers, Sandi quickly recognized that it was the same girl she had assisted in finding a team. She promised the girls that she would look into the matter and issue a ruling the following day.

Sandi contacted North Star Tech's head basketball coach, who verified the girls' claim that Judy had been a member of the varsity team for a few games at the beginning of her freshman year. The coach went on to explain that Judy had been a walk-on player and had played less than 30 minutes total. The coach added that "things just didn't work out" so Judy left the team before mid-season.

In Sandi's mind, this was an open-and-shut case. The intramural rule stated clearly that a walk-on or scholarship player, anyone with previous varsity experience, was ineligible for intramural participation in that sport. Sandi immediately picked up the telephone and called Judy. Sandi explained the rule, and said that Judy would not be eligible to play intramural basketball. She told her, though, that she could take part in any other intramural activities. Judy listened politely and offered no complaint.

The next day, Ms. James received a telephone call from Mr. Allen, the Director of Athletics, requesting a meeting. When she arrived at Mr. Allen's office, Sandi could sense that something was wrong. Mr. Allen began by asking if any rules prohibited a former varsity player from participating in the intramural program. Before Sandi could respond, he began to tell her about a young lady who had played "only a brief time" on the school's varsity team before being dismissed from the team for creating problems among the other players. He went on to explain that the coach was so upset with the girl that she wouldn't even allow her to try out for the team the following year. It came as no surprise to Sandi that the player was none other than Judy Byers.

At that point, Mr. Allen handed Sandi a letter. As she read it, she could hardly believe her eyes. The letter was from Judy Byers' father, a powerful attorney in a nearby city. Although the letter was lengthy, its point was clear. Judy's father was angry that she had been "totally excluded" from playing basketball at North Star Tech and was prepared to go to court to "settle the issue." As Sandi read the letter a second time, Mr. Allen pointed out that it wasn't the first time Mr. Byers had written an "uncomplimentary" letter to the Athletics Department.

As if the letter wasn't enough, Mr. Allen showed Sandi a memo he had just received from the college president, which read, "First she is dropped from the varsity basketball team, and now she can't even play in the intramural program. What is going on over there?"

Mr. Allen then explained that there was nothing he could do to alter the situation in his department and gently pleaded with Sandi to reconsider the eligibility rule for intramural participation — or at least make an exception in this case. After all, he reminded her, the president is sensitive to any unfavorable publicity.

As she walked back to her office, Sandi thought, "Once again, the Athletics Department has dropped a problem in someone else's lap — and now I'm supposed to solve it."

Case Analysis Report Form
21D – North Star Technical College — Anyone For a Little Game of Basketball?

I. Brief Overview:

II. Principal Characters:

III. Essential Facts:

IV. Specific Major Problems:

V. Specific Sub-problems (if any):

VI. Proposed Solutions:

Immediate/Current

Long-Term

VII. Justification:

Case Scenario 21E

Bay View University — Somebody is Responsible!

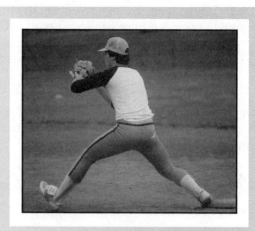

It is a bright, sunny day on the Bay View University campus — a perfect day for intramural softball. All the outdoor playing fields at BVU are the exclusive property of the Athletics Department. Therefore, the Intramural Department rents field space from the Bay View City Recreation Department. The softball fields are 6 miles from campus, but the facilities are great. In addition to two softball fields, the recreation complex has three tennis courts, two outdoor basketball courts, a patio/cookout area, restroom facilities, and a paved parking lot.

On this particular day, three members of the BVU Intramural Department staff gathered up all the necessary equipment, loaded it into a school van, and headed out to the softball fields. This was their favorite part of the day, as they not only enjoyed the camaraderie but also welcomed the opportunity to get away from campus. When they arrived at the field, they quickly put out the bases and prepared for the first game of the afternoon. As game time neared, only one team had arrived at the field. By game time, only two players from the other team had showed up. No one was really surprised by the forfeit, because the losing team

had developed quite a reputation as "no shows."

Having won the game by forfeit, the team that was present soon left the field. Because other games were to follow, the intramural staff members could not leave the site. With nearly an hour until the next game, the three grabbed a basketball from the van and began to shoot a few hoops. Not long after that, the two players from the no show team joined them on the basketball court. Although the level of play was not high, the competition became spirited. While running for a loose ball, Sean, one of the softball players, and Jeff, one of the intramural workers, collided. Sean immediately fell to the ground, clutching his knee.

Jeff offered Sean an ice pack and said he would be glad to drive Sean to the hospital. Sean politely declined, noting that this wasn't the first time he had injured the knee. With Jeff's assistance, Sean made it to his friend's car and left for the hospital.

That night, Jeff telephoned Sean to ask about the injury. To his surprise, Sean's roommate answered the phone and advised Jeff that Sean's injury had required surgery. Stunned, Jeff told the roommate to tell Sean that he had called, then he hung up. Before leaving the Intramural Office, Jeff filled out an injury report.

Several months later, Chris Courtney, BVU's Director of Intramurals, was summoned to the office of Mr. Lake Palmer, the university's Comptroller. As he sat down, Mr. Palmer handed Chris the following letter:

Office of Financial Services
Bay View University
Bay View, USA 12345

Attn: Mr. Lake Palmer, Comptroller

Dear Mr. Palmer:

On April 3 of last year, my son Sean was injured in an intramural-related incident. I present the following account of the events of that day for your consideration.

Sean's intramural softball team was scheduled to play a game at Bay View City Park. However, his team failed to field the required number of players, so a forfeit was declared. The remaining boys, including Sean, organized a basketball game, during which Sean's right knee was seriously injured, resulting in surgery. Following the surgery, Sean was in a brace, on crutches, and in almost constant pain throughout final exam week. Now, nearly seven months later, Sean continues to experience considerable discomfort, and must wear a protective brace for any type of physical activity.

My attempts to get reimbursement from my medical insurance company have been unsuccessful, since the physician who performed Sean's surgery and the hospital where the surgery was done are not "affiliated program providers" for my insurance company. My appeal was recently rejected for the same reason — the use of "non-affiliated providers." The fact that I approved the surgery without first consulting my primary physician apparently negated my insurance coverage. The net result is that the injury has cost me $2,460.39 in out-of-pocket expenses.

Therefore, I am asking that Bay View University provide partial or full reimbursement through the university's insurance plan, since the injury was sustained during intramural-related activities. With two children in college, we simply cannot afford these added expenses.

Sincerely,

Stanford J. Simmons, Jr.
cc: Fred C. Wilson, Atty. at Law

Mr. Palmer told Chris that the university's liability insurance policy provided for a pre-trial settlement of injury complaints in the maximum amount of $1,000. Mr. Palmer indicated that he was leaning in the direction of making such an offer to Mr. Simmons. Chris wasn't sure that was a good idea.

Case Analysis Report Form
21E – Bay View University — Somebody is Responsible!

I. Brief Overview:

II. Principal Characters:

III. Essential Facts:

IV. Specific Major Problems:

V. Specific Sub-problems (if any):

VI. Proposed Solutions:

Immediate/Current

Long-Term

VII. Justification:

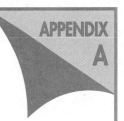

Recommended Format
for a Participation Agreement

**YOU MUST READ AND SIGN THIS AGREEMENT
BEFORE BEING ALLOWED TO PARTICIPATE**

1. Give a general description of the activity. Pay particular attention to the nature of the activity as related to the level of intensity needed to participate in the activity. If the activity is one that is not a more common activity, compare it to a more common activity.

2. If the activity has specific aspects that are hazardous, list them separately and highlight them here. Tell the potential participant about any safety equipment that is required to protect against the particular hazards of this activity. Inform the potential participant that he/she will not be allowed to participate if required safety equipment is not used. It should also be noted that if the equipment is initially used but later discarded, such action will result in the participant's removal from the activity. Any fees paid will be forfeited.

3. If specific practices can be used to help reduce hazards and the likelihood of injury, give them here. It is especially important to list all safety rules of the activity.

4. If there are specific practices that, if used, will increase the likelihood of injury, warn against them here. It should be noted that hazardous behavior on the part of the participant is also grounds for removal from the activity.

5. Inform the participant of the general attire needed for the activity and why not wearing the correct clothing and shoes can create hazards in the activity, if applicable to this activity.

6. Have the potential participant list any health conditions that might affect his/her ability to participate in this activity. Participants with limiting health conditions or those over 35 years of age should be required to get a physician's clearance before participating in vigorous physical activity. If clearance is obtained, attach the clearance to this agreement.

7. Use a standard statement such as the following:

   I have carefully read each statement above. I have had the opportunity to ask questions concerning this document and the nature of the activity to which this document pertains and have had those questions answered satisfactorily. I am aware that any behavior on my part that violates the rules or the recommended method of performance of this activity increases the likelihood of injury. I am confident that I fully know, understand, and appreciate the risks involved in active participation in____(name of activity)____ and I certify that my state of health poses no problems for such participation. I am voluntarily requesting permission to participate.

_____   _____
Signature   Date

United States Constitution
First Ten Amendments
("Bill of Rights") and Section 1
of the 14th Amendment

AMENDMENT I (1791)

Congress shall make no law respecting an establishment of religion, or prohibiting the free exercise thereof; or abridging the freedom of speech, or of the press, or the right of the people peaceably to assemble, and to petition the Government for a redress of grievances.

AMENDMENT II (1791)

A well regulated Militia, being necessary to the security of a free State, the right of the people to keep and bear Arms, shall not be infringed.

AMENDMENT III (1791)

No soldier shall, in time of peace be quartered in any house, without the consent of the Owner, nor in time of war, but in a manner to be prescribed by law.

AMENDMENT IV (1791)

The right of the people to be secure in their persons, houses, papers, and effects, against unreasonable searches and seizures, shall not be violated, and no Warrants shall issue, but upon probable cause, supported by Oath or affirmation, and particularly describing the place to be searched, and the persons or things to be seized.

AMENDMENT V (1791)

No person shall be held to answer for a capital, or otherwise infamous crime, unless on a presentment or indictment of a Grand Jury, except in cases arising in the land or naval forces, or in the Militia, when in actual service in time of War or public danger; nor shall any person be subject for the same offense to be twice put in jeopardy of life or limb; nor shall be compelled in any criminal case to be a witness against himself, nor be deprived of life, liberty, or property, without due process of law; nor shall private property be taken for public use, without just compensation.

AMENDMENT VI (1791)

In all criminal prosecutions, the accused shall enjoy the right to a speedy and public trial, by an impartial jury of the State and district wherein the crime shall have been committed, which district shall have been previously ascertained by law, and to be informed of the nature and cause of the accusation; to be confronted with the witnesses against him; to have compulsory process for obtaining witnesses in his favor, and to have the Assistance of Counsel for his defense.

AMENDMENT VII (1791)

In Suits at common law, where the value in controversy shall exceed twenty dollars, the right of trial by jury shall be reserved, and no fact tried by jury, shall be otherwise re-examined in any Court of the United States, than according to the rules of the common law.

AMENDMENT VIII (1791)

Excessive bail shall not be required, nor excessive fines imposed, nor cruel and unusual punishments inflicted.

AMENDMENT IX (1791)

The enumeration in the Constitution, of certain rights, shall not be construed to deny or disparage others retained by the people.

AMENDMENT X (1791)

The powers not delegated to the United States by the Constitution, nor prohibited by it to the States, are reserved to the States respectively, or to the people.

AMENDMENT XIV (1868)

Section 1. All persons born or naturalized in the United States, and subject to the jurisdiction thereof, are citizens of the United States and of the State wherein they reside. No State shall make or enforce any law which shall abridge the privileges or immunities of citizens of the United States; nor shall any State deprive any person of life, liberty, or property, without due process of law; nor deny to any person within its jurisdiction the equal protection of the laws.

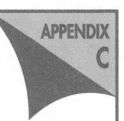
Web Sites

1. **1996** *Surgeon General's Report on Physical Activity and Health*
   http://www.cdc.gov/nccdphp/sgr/intro1.htm
   Contains Chapter 1, the introduction to the Surgeon General's Report. A summary of the
   other chapters and other information is available under the following web site.

2. **Summary of the 1996** *Surgeon General's Report on Physical Activity and Health*
   http://www.cdc.gov/nccdphp/sgr/summary.htm
   The 1996 Surgeon General's Report is a 6,107-page document. This web site gives you
   a statement from the Surgeon General and a summary of the chapters beginning with
   Chapter 2.

3. **Organizational Effectiveness Group**
   http://www.oeg.net

4. **Office of Disease Prevention and Health Promotion Home Page**
   http://www.oeg.net

5. **Sexual Harassment Training**
   http://www.de.psu.edu/harass/intro.htm
   A sexual harassment training module by Nancy Wyatt, Associate Professor of Speech
   Communication and Women's Studies, Delaware County Campus, Penn State University.

6. **Sports Medicine, Athletic Training and Exercise Science Links**
   http://www.mspweb.com
   Links to organizations, schools, publications, clinics, and other points of interest.

7. **National Coalition for Promoting Physical Activity**
   http://www.ncppa.org

8. **American College of Sports Medicine**
   http://www.acsm.org

9. **Association for Worksite Health Promotion**
   http://www.awhp.org

10. **President's Council on Physical Fitness and Sports**
    http://www.os.dhhs.gov/progorg/ophs/pcpfs.htm

11. **Wellness Councils of America**
    http://www.welcoa.org

12. **American Alliance for Health, Physical Education, Recreation and Dance**
    http://www.aahperd.org

13. National Recreation and Park Association
    http://www.nrpa.org

14. National Athletic Trainers' Association
    http://www.nata.org

15. Legal Information Institute at Cornell University
    http://www.law.cornell.edu/lii.html

16. National Alliance for Youth Sports
    http://www.nays.org

17. National Clearinghouse for Youth Sports Information
    http://www.nays.org/ncysi.html

18. Lycos Sports Administration Site
    http://www.lycos.com/cgi-bin/pursuit?cat=point&matchmode=and&query=sports+administration

19. Lycos Law Search Site
    http://point.lycos.com/reviews/Law_12482.html

20. National Intramural-Recreational Sports Association
    http://www.nirsa.org

21. United States Olympic Committee
    http://www.usoc.org

22. Virginia Tech University Physical Education Resource Site
    http://pe.central.vt.edu

23. United States Organization for Disabled Athletes
    http://www.wwgv.com/usoda/

24. National Sports Center for the Disabled
    http://www.nscd.org/nscd/

25. Physical Activity and Disability
    http://info.lut.ac.uk/research/paad/home.html

26. Disabled Sports USA
    http://www.dsusa.org/%7Edsusa/

Index

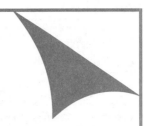